Small Animal Orthopedic Surgery, Physical Therapy and Rehabilitation

Small Animal Orthopedic Surgery, Physical Therapy and Rehabilitation

Guest Editors

L. Miguel Carreira
João Alves

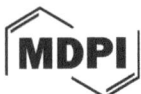

Basel • Beijing • Wuhan • Barcelona • Belgrade • Novi Sad • Cluj • Manchester

Guest Editors

L. Miguel Carreira
Faculty of Veterinary Medicine
University of Lisbon
Lisbon
Portugal

João Alves
Department of Veterinary Medicine
Republican National Guard
Lisbon
Portugal

Editorial Office
MDPI AG
Grosspeteranlage 5
4052 Basel, Switzerland

This is a reprint of the Special Issue, published open access by the journal *Animals* (ISSN 2076-2615), freely accessible at: www.mdpi.com/journal/animals/special_issues/IUK6628V5H.

For citation purposes, cite each article independently as indicated on the article page online and using the guide below:

Lastname, A.A.; Lastname, B.B. Article Title. *Journal Name* **Year**, *Volume Number*, Page Range.

ISBN 978-3-7258-3252-1 (Hbk)
ISBN 978-3-7258-3251-4 (PDF)
https://doi.org/10.3390/books978-3-7258-3251-4

© 2025 by the authors. Articles in this book are Open Access and distributed under the Creative Commons Attribution (CC BY) license. The book as a whole is distributed by MDPI under the terms and conditions of the Creative Commons Attribution-NonCommercial-NoDerivs (CC BY-NC-ND) license (https://creativecommons.org/licenses/by-nc-nd/4.0/).

Contents

About the Editors vii

Preface ix

Nedim Zaimovic, Dragan Lorinson, Karin Lorinson, Alexander Tichy and Barbara Bockstahler
Evaluation of the Tibial Plateau–Patella Angle (TPPA) in Dogs
Reprinted from: *Animals* **2024**, *14*, 1798, https://doi.org/10.3390/ani14121798 1

Sanghyun Nam, Youngjin Jeon, Haebeom Lee and Jaemin Jeong
Effects of the Direction of Two Kirschner Wires on Combined Tibial Plateau Leveling Osteotomy and Tibial Tuberosity Transposition in Miniature Breed Dogs: An Ex Vivo Study
Reprinted from: *Animals* **2024**, *14*, 2258, https://doi.org/10.3390/ani14152258 14

Minji Bae, Byung-Jae Kang and Junhyung Kim
Application of Hybrid External Skeletal Fixation with Bone Tissue Engineering Techniques for Comminuted Fracture of the Proximal Radius in a Dog
Reprinted from: *Animals* **2024**, *14*, 3480, https://doi.org/10.3390/ani14233480 25

Keun-Yung Kim, Minha Oh and Minkyung Kim
Treatment of a Large Tibial Non-Union Bone Defect in a Cat Using Xenograft with Canine-Derived Cancellous Bone, Demineralized Bone Matrix, and Autograft
Reprinted from: *Animals* **2024**, *14*, 690, https://doi.org/10.3390/ani14050690 37

Eunbin Jeong, Youngjin Jeon, Taewan Kim, Dongbin Lee and Yoonho Roh
Assessing the Effectiveness of Modified Tibial Plateau Leveling Osteotomy Plates for Treating Cranial Cruciate Ligament Rupture and Medial Patellar Luxation in Small-Breed Dogs
Reprinted from: *Animals* **2024**, *14*, 1937, https://doi.org/10.3390/ani14131937 47

Jong-Pil Yoon, Hae-Beom Lee, Young-Jin Jeon, Dae-Hyun Kim, Seong-Mok Jeong and Jae-Min Jeong
Reconstruction of Bilateral Chronic Triceps Brachii Tendon Disruption Using a Suture-Mediated Anatomic Footprint Repair in a Dog
Reprinted from: *Animals* **2024**, *14*, 1687, https://doi.org/10.3390/ani14111687 58

Hyunho Kim, Haebeom Lee, Daniel D. Lewis, Jaemin Jeong, Gyumin Kim and Youngjin Jeon
Reconstruction of the Quadriceps Extensor Mechanism with a Calcaneal Tendon–Bone Allograft in a Dog with a Resorbed Tibial Tuberosity Fracture
Reprinted from: *Animals* **2024**, *14*, 2315, https://doi.org/10.3390/ani14162315 68

Joanna Bonecka, Michał Skibniewski, Paweł Zep and Małgorzata Domino
Knee Joint Osteoarthritis in Overweight Cats: The Clinical and Radiographic Findings
Reprinted from: *Animals* **2023**, *13*, 2427, https://doi.org/10.3390/ani13152427 78

J. C. Alves, Ana Santos and L. Miguel Carreira
A Preliminary Report on the Combined Effect of Intra-Articular Platelet-Rich Plasma Injections and Photobiomodulation in Canine Osteoarthritis
Reprinted from: *Animals* **2023**, *13*, 3247, https://doi.org/10.3390/ani13203247 94

Henry G. Spratt, Nicholas Millis, David Levine, Jenna Brackett and Darryl Millis
Bacterial Contamination of Environmental Surfaces of Veterinary Rehabilitation Clinics
Reprinted from: *Animals* **2024**, *14*, 1896, https://doi.org/10.3390/ani14131896 105

About the Editors

L. Miguel Carreira

L. Miguel Carreira holds the following academic degrees: Doctor of Veterinary Medicine, Doctor of Human Medicine in Dentistry, Diploma in Orthopedics and Trauma in Small Animals, postgraduate international training in several veterinary and human medicine and surgery fields, Master's of Science, and Doctorate in Veterinary Sciences (branch of clinic—specialty in surgery with his research focusing on brain neurosurgery and neuronavigation in the dog).

Dr. Carreira has co-authored a series of acclaimed studies and publications on CO_2 laser surgery, particularly on intra- and post-operative pain and post-operative healing. For his contributions, he was awarded the prestigious 2022 World Kumar Patel Prize in Laser Surgery.

Currently, he is an Assistant Professor with the Faculty of Veterinary Medicine—with an Aggregation degree—at the University of Lisbon, teaching surgery, basic and advanced life support, and CO_2 laser surgery (all in small animals). He is both a member and an honorary member of the Faculty of American Laser Study Club—ALSC—in the USA. He is also eligible for membership in the European College of Veterinary Sport Medicine and Rehabilitation—ECVSMR.

He is the Clinical Director of a private referral Veterinary Medicine Centre—Anjos of Assis Veterinary Medicine Centre in Barreiro, Portugal. He has authored numerous scientific papers published in international indexed journals and belongs to the editorial boards of several prestigious human and veterinary medical international journals.

Dr. Carreira's scientific interests in veterinary medicine focus on neurosurgery (brain and medulla), orthopedics/trauma and rehabilitation, plastic surgery, CO_2 laser surgery, anesthesia, pain management, transplantation, and biomaterials for surgery applications. In human dentistry, his interests and research include surgery, implants, and cosmetic dentistry.

João Alves

João Alves graduated from the University of Lisbon, Portugal, in 2012 and has since worked at the Guarda Nacional Republicana (Portuguese Gendarmerie) with their police working dogs, focusing on sports medicine and rehabilitation, helping these animals achieve their full potential. He completed his Ph.D. in 2021 from the University of Évora, Portugal, in intra-articular management modalities for osteoarthritis. In 2022, he became a European Specialist in Canine Sports Medicine and Rehabilitation (Diplomate of the European College of Sports Medicine and Rehabilitation—Small Animals; DECVSMR). In addition to osteoarthritis, he carries out research and is interested in working dog sports medicine, photobiomodulation therapy, and canine exercise. João has published dozens of papers and lectures on these topics.

Preface

The fields of small animal orthopedic surgery, physical therapy, and rehabilitation have undergone remarkable advancements, transforming the management of musculoskeletal conditions. This Special Issue is dedicated to exploring these innovations, highlighting collaborative research and practical applications aiming to enhance the quality of life for small animal patients.

Orthopedic conditions are common challenges. Addressing these issues demands a multidisciplinary approach. Innovations in minimally invasive techniques, such as arthroscopy, and the development of patient-specific implants through 3D printing have revolutionized surgical outcomes. Moreover, regenerative therapies offer promising avenues for restoring joint health and addressing chronic conditions.

Rehabilitation has also become a cornerstone of comprehensive orthopedic care. Evidence-based protocols are now integral to post-surgical recovery and the management of chronic conditions. These therapies not only accelerate recovery but also enhance mobility, particularly in aging animals or those with long-standing musculoskeletal challenges.

Articles featured in this Special Issue reflect the depth and breadth of progress in small animal orthopedic care. Studies include innovative approaches to planning patellar luxation surgeries, advancements in tibial plateau-leveling osteotomies, and biomechanical evaluations of implant techniques for complex cases. Additionally, novel surgical interventions, such as the reconstruction of the quadriceps extensor mechanism and triceps brachii tendon, underscore the ingenuity required to address unique clinical presentations. Research on the effects of photobiomodulation and platelet-rich plasma on osteoarthritis and the impact of obesity on joint health further emphasizes the importance of preventive and therapeutic strategies in improving outcomes.

Beyond clinical techniques, this Special Issue highlights critical considerations in the area of broader care, with research on bacterial contamination in rehabilitation clinics underscoring the importance of maintaining hygienic practices to safeguard patient health. Together, these studies represent a cohesive effort addressing the multifaceted challenges of small animal orthopedic and rehabilitation care.

The future of this field is promising, with continued advancements poised to redefine standards of care, ultimately improving the lives of companion animals worldwide.

We extend our gratitude to the authors who contributed their expertise, the reviewers who ensured the rigor of the studies, and MDPI's editorial and management teams for their dedication to presenting this collection. This Special Issue serves as both a reflection of progress and a call to action for further exploration and innovation in small animal orthopedics, physical therapy, and rehabilitation. Together, we can ensure that our patients lead healthier, more active, and pain-free lives.

L. Miguel Carreira and João Alves
Guest Editors

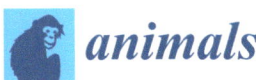

Article

Evaluation of the Tibial Plateau–Patella Angle (TPPA) in Dogs

Nedim Zaimovic [1,*], Dragan Lorinson [2], Karin Lorinson [2], Alexander Tichy [3] and Barbara Bockstahler [4]

1. Small Animal Surgery, Department for Companion Animals and Horses, University of Veterinary Medicine, 1210 Vienna, Austria
2. Chirurgisches Zentrum für Kleintiere Dr. Lorinson, 2331 Vösendorf, Austria; ordination@vet-lorinson.com (D.L.); karinunddragan@hotmail.com (K.L.)
3. Platform Bioinformatics and Biostatistics, Department for Biomedical Services, University of Veterinary Medicine, 1120 Vienna, Austria; alexander.tichy@vetmeduni.ac.at
4. Section of Physical Therapy, Small Animal Surgery, Department for Companion Animals and Horses, University of Veterinary Medicine, 1210 Vienna, Austria; barbara.bockstahler@vetmeduni.ac.at
* Correspondence: nedim.zaimovic@vetmeduni.ac.at

Simple Summary: The proximodistal patellar position in canine pathologies, including patella luxation, cruciate ligament rupture, and osteoarthrosis, is not fully understood, while this topic is much better understood in human medicine. Various methods are used to confirm the proximodistal patellar position, but they all require calculations and are infrequently used in everyday practice. In a two-step study with three observers, we investigated, for the first time in veterinary medicine, the applicability of a new, simple method derived from human medicine called the tibial plateau–patella angle (TPPA). This method is independent of the knee angle and magnification, does not require any calculations, and consists of just two lines. This study started with cadavers at different stifle angles. Subsequently, we used 100 X-rays at the optimal stifle angle based on these findings. In both study phases, our results revealed strong agreement among observers. The TPPA varied with the stifle angle but remained consistent across the different weight groups. We concluded that the TPPA is directly dependent on the stifle angulation and tends to be lower with a higher stifle extension angle. It could be difficult for some observers to establish the exact caudal border of the tibial plateau while measuring the TPPA. While the TPPA method shows promise, further evaluation, including breed-specific and pathological considerations, is necessary.

Citation: Zaimovic, N.; Lorinson, D.; Lorinson, K.; Tichy, A.; Bockstahler, B. Evaluation of the Tibial Plateau–Patella Angle (TPPA) in Dogs. *Animals* **2024**, *14*, 1798. https://doi.org/10.3390/ani14121798

Academic Editors: L. Miguel Carreira and João Alves

Received: 7 May 2024
Revised: 7 June 2024
Accepted: 11 June 2024
Published: 16 June 2024

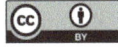

Copyright: © 2024 by the authors. Licensee MDPI, Basel, Switzerland. This article is an open access article distributed under the terms and conditions of the Creative Commons Attribution (CC BY) license (https://creativecommons.org/licenses/by/4.0/).

Abstract: Estimating a dog's patellar position involves various methods, which categorize it as norma, alta (high), or baja (low). However, they require various calculations. We aimed to evaluate the clinical applicability of a new method, the tibial plateau–patella angle (TPPA). This could aid in planning patella luxation surgery, estimating the patella position after TPLO and various osteotomies. We conducted a two-step study: first, on 15 stifles without pathologies from nine canine cadavers, and second, using 100 patient X-rays from the archive. Three stifle angle positions (45 ± 5°, 90 ± 5°, and 135 ± 5°) and three weight groups (S, M, and L) were evaluated in the first part of this study. Based on these results, the second part of this study was conducted using 100 pathology-free radiographs at the optimal stifle angle (90 ± 5°) from the archive. All radiographs were measured by three observers with varying levels of experience. Our results indicate that the stifle angle significantly impacted the TPPA, whereby lower values were detected with higher stifle angles, which remained consistent within the weight groups. High inter- and intra-observer agreement was achieved. The physiological TPPA values ranged from 26.7° to 48.8°, remaining consistent within the various weight groups. Observer 3 in Group S exhibited a 20% (insignificant) deviation, possibly due to challenges in determining the caudal point of the tibial plateau. In contrast with humans, TPPA values in dogs are negatively correlated with stifle angles, independent of weight. Our reliable and reproducible protocol suggests the potential benefits of training on small-breed dogs stifles.

Keywords: TPPA; proximodistal patellar position; radiography; joint angulation; dog

1. Introduction

The patella is the largest sesamoid bone, sliding in the femoral trochlea, and is crucial to the biomechanics of the stifle joint. Patellar luxation is one of the most common stifle joint pathologies in dogs. Medial patellar luxation is more frequent and classified as congenital, developmental, or traumatic. The underlying issue is not precisely understood; however, most patients show structural abnormalities [1–3]. Cranial cruciate ligament disease and patellar luxation, the most common clinical stifle conditions in dogs, lead to the development of osteoarthrosis [4,5]. The influence of the patellar height on clinical pathologies in canines is not precisely defined.

None of the most commonly used indices are ideal for measuring the proximodistal position of the patella [6]. In human medicine, the impact of the patellar height is much more thoroughly researched. For instance, it is known that patella alta can be responsible for stifle pain, patellofemoral instability, a reduced range of motion, and reduced long-term implant survival (total stifle arthroplasty) [7–12]. Patella alta is also associated with Osgood–Schlatter disease, a painful patellofemoral syndrome in humans [13–15]. In humans, patella baja is a common cause of osteoarthritis (OA) in the patellofemoral joint and represents a significant complication following stifle surgeries, traumas, or immobilization. It can also lead to the shortening of the patellar tendon, fibrosis of the infrapatellar fat pad, intra-articular adhesions, etc. Patella baja is a component of infrapatellar contracture syndrome (IPCS), where the lowering of the patella results from scarring due to inflammation in the peripatellar fat pad, triggered by trauma from surgery [16,17]. Patellofemoral OA is a more common cause of pain in the front of the knee than OA in the tibiofemoral joint [18]. In an experimental study on rats, Bei et al. [19] demonstrated that patella baja may be responsible for the development of osteoarthritic changes.

Radiography is the most common imaging method for orthopedic assessments in small animal practice. Radiological determination of the proximodistal patellar position can be complicated by factors such as osteophytes, joint effusion, an unusual patellar morphology, abnormalities in the tibial tuberosity, and an atypical distal attachment of the patellar tendon [7,20–23].

In veterinary medicine, several studies have evaluated patellar height in dogs. The most commonly used methods for determining patellar height include the (modified) Insall–Salvati index (ISI) [24–27], the Blackburne–Peel index (BPI) [6,26], the de Carvalho index (CDI) [6], the ratio of the patellar ligament length (PLL) to the patellar length (PL) (PLL:PL or L:P), and the ratio of the distance from the proximal aspect of the patella (A) to the femur condyle and patellar length (PL) (A:PL) [21,22,28].

In 2011, Portner and Pakzad [29] developed the tibial plateau–patella angle (TPPA) for determining patellar height, aiming for it to be independent of human knee angle. The measurement is conducted on a mediolateral X-ray knee image (with a minimum flexion of 30°). The advantages of this method include easy reproducibility, no need for calculations, independence from magnification errors, and the degree of limb flexion [29], making it a simple and fast way to determine the proximodistal patellar position in everyday practice. TPPA measurements in dogs have been performed to compare the pre- and post-operative outcomes in TPLO and TTA patients, but without knowledge of its physiological range [26].

Previous studies in dogs have found that an L:P ratio of >1.97–2.06 or an A:PL ratio of >2.03 indicates patella alta [21,22,28]. Patella alta is highly prevalent in German Shepherd dogs, even without a relevant stifle joint pathology; however, these dogs have twice the risk of developing canine hip dysplasia [25]. Unlike in large dogs, the PLL:PL ratios in small dogs without a stifle joint pathology and with patellar luxation showed no significant difference. According to this study, assessing the proximodistal patellar position using only the PLL:PL ratio may not be feasible [30]. In two different studies, it was concluded that small-breed dogs with medial patellar luxation did not have a proximally positioned patella compared with a control group without medial patellar luxation [30,31].

In Figure 1, we present a simplified scheme of the most commonly used methods for dog stifle measurement, compared to the TPPA.

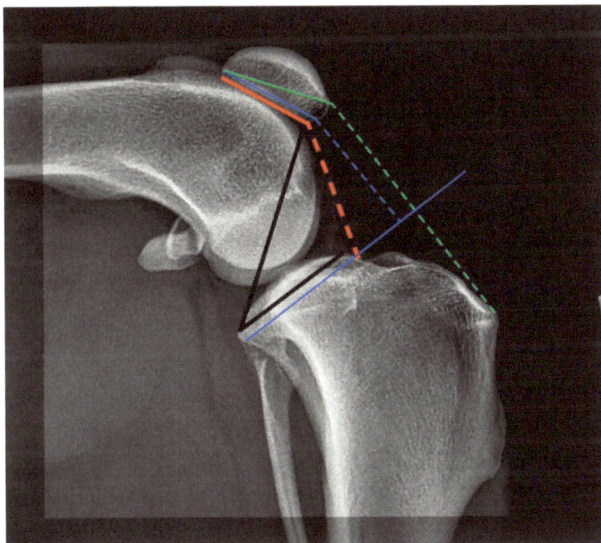

Figure 1. Simplified schematic presentation of the most commonly used indices for estimating patellar height on a dog's stifle. Green lines represent the Insall–Salvati index (ISI: Solid line = patellar length; Dash line = patellar ligament lenght); red lines represent the de Carvalho index (CDI: Solid line = articular patellar length; Dash line = distance from distal articular surface to closest tibial cortex); blue lines represent the Blackburne–Peel index (BPI: proximal Solid line: articular patellar length; Dash line and distal Solid line: perpendicular distance to the distal articular surface from a line extended along the tibial plateau), black lines represent the tibial plateau–patella angle (TPPA: a detailed description follows in this study).

Since the TPPA in dogs has not been previously described and there is no available evidence for observer reliability, we intended to establish the TPPA as a reliable measurement method for assessing patellar height in dogs. We divided this study into two parts: part one involved a cadaver study, and part two involved a patient study.

In the first part of this study, we aimed to evaluate the impact of the stifle angle on the TPPA, examine observer influence, evaluate the influence of body weight, and determine the optimal stifle angle for measuring the TPPA. The second aim was to evaluate whether observers could reliably identify all the important anatomical points for TPPA measurements.

The main goals of the second part of this study were to measure the TPPA at the optimal stifle angle, establish a physiological range, assess the impact of body weight on TPPA values, and control the identification of anatomical measuring points. We hypothesized that the stifle angulation would influence the TPPA in dogs and both inter- and intra-observer variability would be low. Due to its easy applicability, this method may be useful in everyday practice, such as establishing a normal or pathological patellar height in the pre-operative planning of patellar luxation surgery or the insertion of a stifle endoprosthesis.

2. Study Part One: Cadaver Study

2.1. Materials and Methods

The first part of this study was a cadaver study that provided TPPA measurements of 15 canine stifle joints derived from 9 dog cadavers. The dogs were euthanized for reasons unrelated to our study. The cadavers were fresh and free from stifle pathologies. To ensure this, after euthanasia, each cadaver stifle was clinically examined for the persistence of joint effusion, crepitations, cranial/caudal cruciate ligament rupture, patellar luxation, or medial and lateral stifle joint instability. After a stifle was found to be compatible with these criteria, we performed control radiographs (craniocaudal and mediolateral) to rule out malalignments, malformations, or osteoarthrosis. If any of these abnormalities (clinical or radiographic) were persistent, the cadaveric stifle was excluded from this study. We obtained written approval from the owner for every cadaver used.

Based on body weight, three different weight groups were defined (S—small: <15 kg, M—medium: ≥15–<30 kg, and L—large: ≥30 kg). Six of the dog cadavers were females (three spayed), and three were males (two castrated). Four dog cadavers (six stifles) belonged to the S weight group, two (three stifles) to M, and three (six stifles) to L. The mean age of the dog cadavers was 9.1 ± 2.8 (range: 4–13) years.

Mediolateral X-rays at three different angles (45°, 90°, and 135°) were performed on each stifle, with a tolerance level of 5°. The ~45° (40–50°) angulation was defined as Group 1, ~90° (85–95°) as Group 2, and 135° (130–140°) as Group 3. The angulation was directly measured on the cadavers during positioning using a goniometer and later verified in the digital X-ray images using the angle function. All the radiographs provided a clear identification of the relevant anatomical points. The 45 X-rays were numerically anonymized. In this study, the authors agreed that a measurement difference between observers of ±5° was negligible and should not significantly impact the final results or, for example, the decision on surgical intervention. The angle consists of two lines. The distal line is drawn tangentially to the tibial plateau, extending from its cranial point to its most caudal point. The proximal line is drawn from the distal margin of the patellar articular surface to the caudal point of the distal line on the tibial plateau (Figure 2) [32].

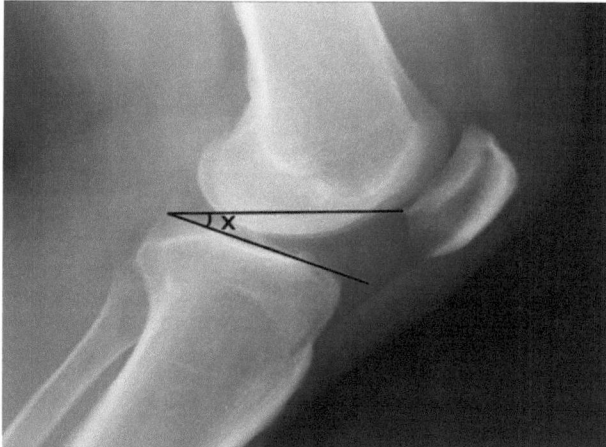

Figure 2. Two lines (distal and proximal) forming the TPPA in human knee.

Establishing the anatomical reference points on a dog stifle was a key factor when conducting this study. The tibial plateau was determined using the conventional Slocum method [33,34]. The tibial plateau was measured as a tangent to the medial tibial plateau comparable to the TPLO measurements (cranial to caudal point of plateau), strictly parallel to the tibial epiphyseal line [26,29]. We established the long axis of the tibia by connecting a line from the tibial intercondylar eminence to the center of the talar body.

The resulting TPPA was automatically calculated and documented as the TPPA measurement (Figure 3).

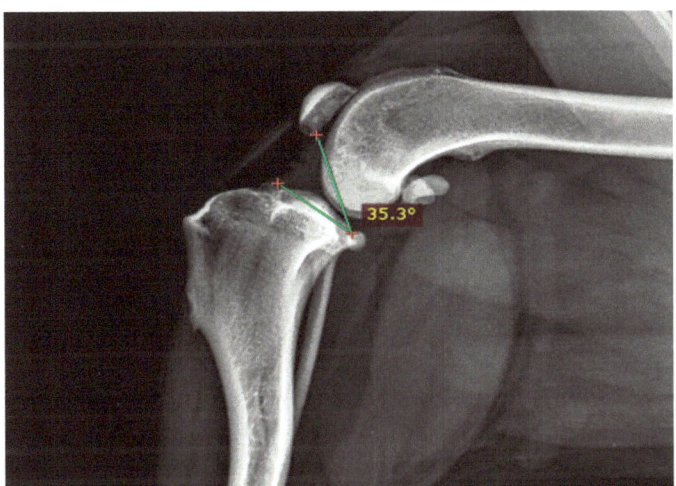

Figure 3. The distal line indicates the tibial plateau from its most cranial to its most caudal point. The proximal line extends from the caudal end of the tibial plateau to the distal end of the patellar articular surface.

Three observers with varying levels of experience measured the TPPAs (using Portner and Pakzad's method (2011) [29]) in the randomized X-rays in random order, twice and one month apart. Before commencing the measurements, all three observers underwent training on the anatomical points in various stifle X-rays.

One of the three observers was a young veterinarian with 4 years of experience in veterinary medicine (O1), another was an ECVS diplomate with over 30 years of surgical experience (O2), and the third had completed a surgical residency, with over 15 years of experience in imaging diagnostics (O3). The measurements were performed with RadiAnt™ DICOM Viewer (Version Nr: 5.0.2.21911, Copyright C 2009–2022 Medixant, Poznan, Poland) using the angle function.

2.2. Statistical Analysis

All the statistical analyses were performed using IBM SPSS v.27. Confirmation of a normal distribution was assessed using the Kolmogorov–Smirnov test. Besides descriptive statistics, we analyzed the agreement between the first and second TPPA measurements for every observer using the dependent-samples *t*-test. We used the interclass correlation coefficient (ICC) to determine the correlations between observers and analyze the agreement between the three observers regarding different stifle angles, weights, and the TPPA (Groups 1, 2, and 3). We used a mixed model to analyze the TPPA in the first and second measurement rounds for the different stifle angles and weight groups and to compare the differences within the stifle angle and weight groups. ANOVA was used to determine the correlations between the different stifle angles and weight groups. A *p*-value below 5% ($p < 0.05$) was considered significant for all the statistical analyses. A difference of ±5° between observers was not considered significant.

2.3. Results of the Cadaver Study

The tibial plateau–patella angle (TPPA) significantly differed between the three stifle angle groups ($p < 0.001$). The mean TPPA was 40.61 ± 4.21° in Group 1 (45°), 35.18 ± 4.21° in Group 2 (90°), and 27.92 ± 4.21° in Group 3 (135°). Figure 4 presents the TPPA measurement at various stifle angles.

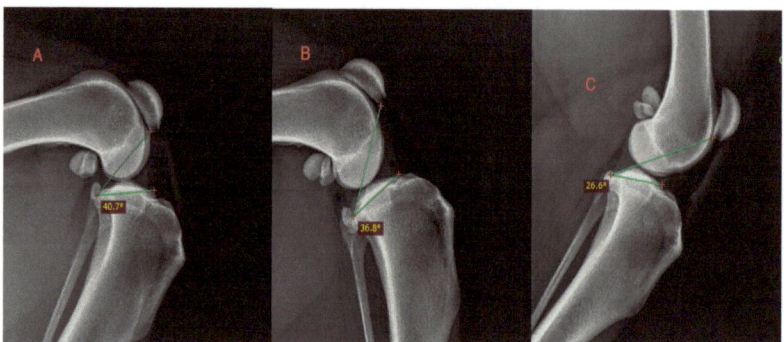

Figure 4. TPPA measurement at various stifle angles. (**A**) 45°; (**B**) 90°; (**C**) 135°.

Group 1 exhibited significant differences compared with Group 2 ($p = 0.002$); Group 2 differed from Group 3 ($p = 0.001$); and there was a significant difference between Groups 1 and 3 ($p = 0.001$). The higher the stifle angle, the lower the TPPA. The inter-observer agreement was high ($r = 0.852$; $p < 0.001$). Moreover, the intra-observer agreement was high for the first ($r = 0.931$; $p < 0.001$), second ($r = 0.876$; $p < 0.001$), and third ($r = 0.899$; $p < 0.001$) observer. Observers 2 and 3 did not show a significant difference between the first and second measurements. The first observer showed a significant difference between their first and second measurements ($r = 0.8769$; $p = 0.017$), but it still fell within the tolerance range of ±5°. Nevertheless, the overall correlation for the first and second measurements across the three observers was not significant and showed a difference of SD ± 3.07°. The inter- and intra-observer variability was not statistically significant. The TPPA values decreased with a higher stifle angulation for all three observers (Figure 5).

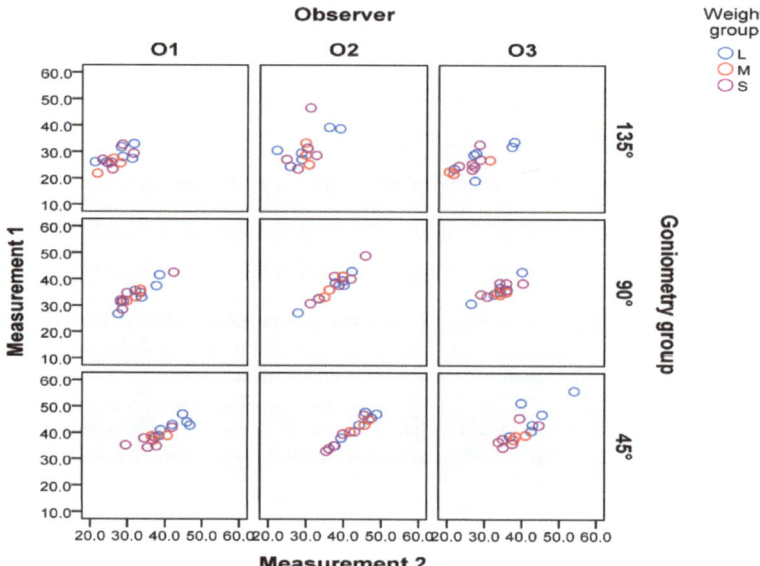

Figure 5. Measurements 1 and 2 across stifle angle and weight groups for all three observers. Values are presented in degrees on the vertical and diagonal axes. The reduction in TPPA values with higher stifle angulation is obvious and consistent across all three observers. Goniometry = stifle angle.

The various stifle angle groups did not influence the measurements across all three observers. Furthermore, the weight group did not have an impact on the measurements by the observers. The measurements in the first and second rounds across the different stifle angles are presented in Figure 5. Body weight did not significantly ($p = 0.347$) influence the mean TPPA in any stifle angle group across all observers. The TPPA values across different weight groups and various stifle angles are presented in Figure 6 and Table 1. None of the groups showed significant variations in the mean TPPA values across the different stifle angle and weight groups. Specifically, the mean TPPA was 40.68° (SD ± 4.28°) in Group 1 (45 ± 5°); 35.26° (SD ± 3.88°) in Group 2 (90 ± 5°); and 28.23° (SD ± 3.54°) in Group 3 (135 ± 5°) (Table 1).

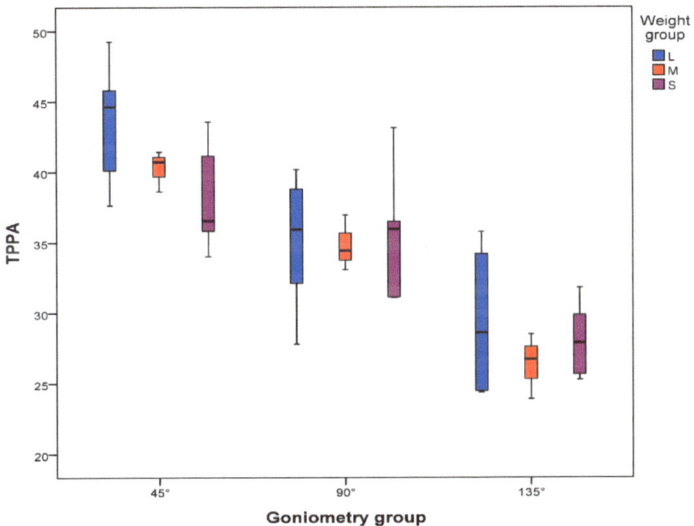

Figure 6. The TPPA in relation to the stifle and weight groups. The TPPA values are presented in degrees. Goniometry = stifle angle.

Table 1. Different weight groups across various stifle angles.

Weight Group	Stifle Angle	Mean TPPA	±SD [1]
~45°	L	43.67°	
	M	40.28°	
	S	37.92°	
Across groups [2]		**40.68°**	**±4.28°**
~90°	L	35.12°	
	M	34.80°	
	S	35.62°	
Across groups		**35.26°**	**±3.88°**
~135°	L	29.32°	
	M	26.37°	
	S	28.06°	
Across groups		**28.23°**	**±3.54°**

[1] Standard deviation. [2] Mean TPPA across stifle angle groups.

3. Study Part Two: Patient Study

3.1. Materials and Methods

In this part of the study, we analyzed archival radiographs based on the influence of the stifle angle on the TPPA in the cadaver study. We chose a positioning of 90 ± 5° because it is the most commonly used clinical projection for stifle joint diagnostics and has excellent inter- and intra-observer reliability. We applied the same inclusion and exclusion criteria as in the cadaver study. For instance, if a dog presented with hind leg lameness and we diagnosed cranial cruciate ligament rupture on one side, we utilized the radiograph of the contralateral (healthy) side for our measurements. We found the radiographs from previous examinations in our archive on optimal angulation and then checked our medical records to determine whether the patient had any current clinical stifle abnormalities. Additionally, a few radiographs from patients exhibited questionable tarsal or hip joint pathologies at the optimal stifle joint angle, allowing us to use both sides for our study. All these radiographs had to meet the same criteria as in the cadaver study to be included in the measurement process.

Therefore, 100 canine stifle radiographs with an angulation of 90 ± 5° were measured to evaluate the physiological limits of the TPPA. A total of 71 dogs were identified in the 100 X-rays, including 37 females (25 spayed) and 34 males (19 neutered). Of the 100 X-rays, 38 belonged to weight Group S, 24 to Group M, and 38 to Group L. The mean ± SD age of the dogs was 6.07 ± 3.5 years (1–13 years). The 100 X-rays from the archive were anonymized and measured in a randomized order once by the same three observers. As in the cadaver study, we allowed a difference of ±5° between observers because we believed this difference would not influence the results of surgical planning. We measured the radiographs under the same conditions and used the same weight categorization as in the cadaver study.

3.2. Statistical Analysis

We employed the ICC, Pearson's correlation coefficient for the inter-observer agreement, and descriptive statistics to analyze the 100 radiographs. We used a mixed model to establish the relationships between observers and different weight groups. We used the same parameters as in the cadaver study. Moreover, we analyzed how many radiographic measurements exceeded the tolerance range of ±5° between observers within different weight groups for a more in-depth understanding.

3.3. Results of the Patient Study

The TPPA measurements in all 71 dogs (100 radiographs) at stifle angulation of 90 ± 5° ranged from 26.7° to 48.8° (Figure 7). The average TPPA for each observer (±SD) is presented in Table 2 and Figure 7.

Table 2. Average TPPA with ±SD for each observer.

Observer	Mean TPPA	±SD
1	36.22°	±4.52°
2	37.10°	±5.29°
3	39.37°	±4.66°

The inter-observer agreement was high (r = 0.861; $p < 0.001$). The correlation between each pair of observers—Observers 1 and 2 (r = 0.858; $p < 0.001$), Observers 1 and 3 (r = 0.890; $p < 0.001$), and Observers 2 and 3 (r = 0.856; $p < 0.001$)—was also substantial.

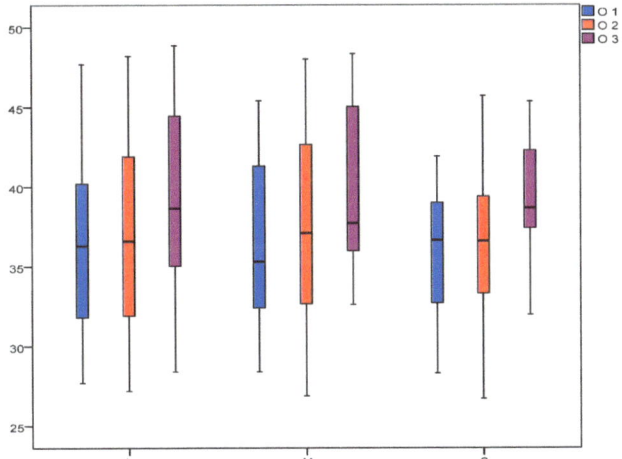

Figure 7. The range of TPPA values across three observers in different weight groups. TPPA values in degrees are presented on the vertical axis, and different weight groups are shown on the horizontal axis. Observer 1 (O1) is presented in blue, Observer 2 (O2) in red, and Observer 3 (O3) in purple.

This difference could also be observed when comparing how many of the 100 X-ray measurements between observers exceeded the tolerance range of ±5°. Just four (4%) radiographs of the 100 X-rays measured by Observers 1 and 2 exceeded the tolerance range of ±5° (one in Group L, two in Group M, and one in Group S). The difference was 14 out of 100 (14%) between Observers 1 and 3 (5 in Group L, 4 in Group M, and 5 in Group S). The largest difference of 20 out of 100 (20%) was observed between Observers 2 and 3 (6 in Group L, 4 in Group M, and 10 in Group S). Generally, the results did not significantly deviate from the tolerance range of ±5°. The variations in the differences between each observer and the mean deviations (MDs) are presented in Table 3.

Table 3. Variations and mean deviations (MDs) between three observers.

Observer	Observer	Difference	MD
1	2	3.62–4.69°	4.15°
1	3	1.48–2.34°	1.95°
2	3	2.21–3.29°	2.75°

4. Discussion

In this study, we aimed to investigate the influence of difference stifle angle groups on the TPPA, establish the physiological TPPA value range in dogs, and assess the inter- and intra-observer reliability of the measurements within various stifle angle and weight groups.

The TPPA values significantly changed at various stifle angles. Compared with studies in humans, different stifle angle groups significantly influenced the TPPA in dogs. This negative correlation (the lower the stifle angle, the higher the TPPA) was consistent and confirmed by all three observers. This can probably be explained by the greater distance between the tibial plateau and the patella at a lower stifle angle. We confirmed our hypothesis that the TPPA in dogs, unlike humans, depends on the stifle angulation.

Obtaining a high-quality radiograph without condylar overlay can be challenging in the 45° stifle position. It is often necessary to capture multiple radiographs to achieve an ideal image.

The patellar height position changes in relation to different tibial plateau angulations, and it has been suggested that a reduction in the tibial plateau increases the load on the patellar ligament. Consequently, the risk of patellar fractures increases as the tibia plateau angle decreases after TPLO [35].

In another study, different stifle angles (75°, 96°, 113°, 130°, and 148°) did not influence the measurements of the PLL-to-PL ratio [31], unlike our TPPA measurements. This represents a significant advantage of the PLL–PL ratio over TPPA measurements because angulation is not a limiting factor.

In a study on human stifles published in 2016, the TPPA was compared with other measurement methods such as the Insall–Salvati (I/S), Caton–Deschamps (C/D), and Blackburne–Peel (B/P) indices [32]. The results indicate that the TPPA values are consistent with those obtained using other methods but change if the surgery includes a tibial slope. Capkin and colleagues [36] reached the same conclusion when comparing the TPPA with the Insall–Salvati, modified Insall–Salvati, Blackburne–Peel, and Caton–Deschamps indices. The TPPA demonstrated higher reliability than the other methods.

The TPPA was pre- and post-operatively evaluated in dogs undergoing TPLO and tibial tuberosity advancement (TTA). The TPPA inconsistently correlated with the Insall–Salvati and Blackburne–Peel indices [26]. The main disadvantage of the study was the absence of a control group and a physiological TPPA value.

The TPPA in the dogs' stifles showed a negative correlation with the Insall–Salvati index but a positive correlation with the differences in the Blackburne–Peel index. It is difficult to compare our results with those of this study because we lack information about the stifle angle in each case [37].

In another study, the proximodistal BPI, ISI, and CDI did not reliably distinguish between healthy stifle joints and joints with medial patellar luxation in small-breed dogs [38].

Small-breed dogs with second-grade medial patellar luxation had a more proximally positioned patellar ligament insertion compared to the control group. This is also a cause of the more proximally positioned patella in the femoral trochlea and probably plays an important role in the pathology of medial patellar luxation [39].

Unfortunately, there is no evidence of pathological TPPA values in dogs, so we can hardly direct compare our results with other studies on the proximodistal patella position.

The physiological TPPA values in our study ranged from 26.7° to 48.8°, with a mean value of 37.75° and MD of ±11.05°. We estimated the physiological TPPA range via our patient study in the 90 ± 10° stifle position. Based on these values, we postulate that angles below 26.7° could be classified as patella baja and angles above 48.8° as patella alta.

In her master's thesis in 2019 [37], Winkler compared the pre- and post-operative (TPLO and TTA) TPPA, Insall–Salvati, and Blackburne–Peel indices in 39 different-sized dogs. She noted changes in the TPPA pre- and post-operatively, with the TPPA values ranging from 14.6° to 45.5° pre-operatively and from 14.6° to 51.4° post-operatively. This difference in the TPPA range may be explained by the cranial cruciate ligament or the low level of experience of one observer who performed the measurements. In Winkler's study, the stifle angle ranged from 30° to 90° and did not influence the evaluation of the TPPA. The TPPA post-TPLO was higher in 35 dogs and lower in 4 dogs. This may have been due to the reduction in the TPA. The TPPA post-TTA was lower in 36 dogs and higher in 4 dogs. However, Winkler concluded that TPLO increases and TTA surgery decreases the TPPA value post-operatively.

Like our study on dogs, a study on the TPPA in cat stifles confirmed that an increasing stifle extension results in a reduction in the TPPA [40]. Our analysis indicates that the TPPA measurements were reproducible for all three observers, and they exhibited strong correlations and reproducibility in the cadaver and patient studies.

The stifle angle group did not influence the reproducibility of the TPPA measurements. As such, the observers could identify all three important anatomical points for measuring the TPPA at different stifle joint angles, but its value changed.

Only the third observer showed a significant difference of ±0.9° between the first and second measurements. However, considering our tolerance range of ±5°, this difference was not considered significant. This deviation in the third observer could be explained by them having less experience than Observers 1 and 2.

The key to obtaining correct and reproducible measurements was the exact identification of all three anatomical points: 1. The cranial edge of the tibial plateau, 2. the caudal tibial plateau, and 3. the distal end of the articular patellar surface. In our experience, the main difficulty is establishing the caudal point of the tibial plateau, where disagreement leads to differences in the TPPA measurements.

The second observer exhibited fewer differences in their measurements than the first and third observers. This could be attributed to the second observer's higher experience level in establishing landmarks on the tibial plateau, as seen in tasks such as planning TPLO (tibial plateau leveling osteotomy) surgery. Determining the proximodistal patellar position can be complicated by factors such as osteophytes, an unusual patellar morphology, and an atypical distal attachment of the patellar ligament [14,20,22,30,41].

The examinations in the patient study revealed no significant differences between the observers, considering our tolerance range of ±5°. Observer 3 continuously measured higher angles than Observers 1 and 2. Observer 3 showed a larger deviation in the S group, which could be because anatomical deformities occur more often in small-breed dogs [3,42] or because the observer experienced more difficulty in identifying the caudal border of the tibial plateau in small-breed dogs. We consistently remained within our tolerance range, demonstrating the reproducibility of the TPPA measurements by the independent observers.

Evaluations of the TPPA in humans also revealed high inter- and intra-observer reliability [29,32,36].

In our experience, we can rely on measurements made by a single observer; however, additional training in small-breed dogs could be beneficial for precisely establishing anatomical points.

All the observers produced consistent TPPA measurements in the different weight groups (S, M, and L) without significant deviations; therefore, weight did not influence the identification of anatomical points. This is important for establishing future studies, for example, on breed-specific TPPA values. No difficulties in detecting the anatomical landmarks for the TPPA in humans have been reported, but poor-quality radiographs were also excluded from study [29].

Considering weight, the TPPA in the cadaver study did not change in relation to the S, M, or L groups. The small deviation in Group M could be due to the very small number of patients in this group (20%). The statistically visible variation in the S group could be explained by the larger deviation in the measurements performed by Observer 3.

Future studies should explore whether the TPPA is reliable for distinguishing between dogs with patellar luxation, cranial cruciate ligament rupture, and normal stifles. One possibility is to evaluate breed-specific TPPA values, particularly in small-breed dogs. A larger sample could allow us to analyze whether taking TPPA measurements in low-weight dogs are more challenging. These studies should compare the physiological reliability of the TPPA with that of other measurement methods.

5. Conclusions

Unlike in a human stifle, the TPPA varies at different stifle angles in dogs. The physiological range of the TPPA spans from 26.7° to 48.8°. The protocol for measuring the TPPA was proven to be reliable and reproducible for various observers. The observer's level of experience may influence the achievement of precise TPPA measurements. Weight is not a significant factor for the successful measurement of the TPPA. Some observers may experience difficulty in establishing the caudal point of the tibial plateau in small-breed dogs.

Author Contributions: Conceptualization, N.Z. and K.L.; methodology, N.Z., B.B., K.L., D.L. and A.T.; validation, N.Z., B.B., K.L., D.L. and A.T.; formal analysis, N.Z. and A.T.; investigation, N.Z., K.L. and D.L.; resources, N.Z., K.L. and D.L.; data curation, N.Z., K.L. and D.L.; writing—original draft preparation, N.Z. and K.L.; writing—review and editing, N.Z., K.L., D.L., B.B. and A.T.; visualization, N.Z., K.L., D.L., B.B. and A.T.; supervision, B.B.; project administration, N.Z. All authors have read and agreed to the published version of the manuscript.

Funding: This research received no external funding. Open Access Funding by the University of Veterinary Medicine Vienna.

Institutional Review Board Statement: The study was conducted in accordance with the Declaration of Helsinki. There are described therapies for anomalies. This case was special due to ectrodactyly in combination with polydactyly. It was not an experiment, so it does not need ethical approval.

Informed Consent Statement: For every cadaver used, we obtained written approval from the owner.

Data Availability Statement: The raw data supporting the conclusions of this article will be made available by the authors on request.

Acknowledgments: All of the cadavers and radiographic images used in this article were from "Chirurgisches Zentrum für Kleintiere Dr. Lorinson". The authors are grateful to Elisabeth Branka and Jana Auer for helping with conducting the radiographs.

Conflicts of Interest: The authors declare no conflicts of interest.

References

1. LaFond, E.; Breuer, G.J.; Austin, C.C. Breed susceptibility for developmental orthopedic diseases in dog. *J. Am. Anim. Hosp. Assoc.* **2002**, *38*, 467–477. [CrossRef]
2. L'Eplattenier, H.; Montavon, P.M. Patellar luxation in dogs and cats: Management and prevention. *Compe. Conti. Educ. Pract. Vet.* **2002**, *24*, 292–298.
3. Roush, J.K. Canine patellar luxation. *Vet. Clin. N. Am. Small Anim. Pract.* **1993**, *23*, 855–868. [CrossRef] [PubMed]
4. Gilbert, S.; Langenbach, A.; Marcellin-Little, D.J.; Pease, A.P.; Ru, H. Stifle joint osteoarthritis at the time of diagnosis of cranial cruciate ligament injury is higher in Boxers and in dogs weighing more than 35 kilograms. *Vet. Radiol. Ultrasound* **2019**, *60*, 280–288. [CrossRef] [PubMed]
5. Roy, R.G.; Wallace, L.J.; Johnston, G.R.; Wickstrom, S.L. A retrospective evaluation of stifle osteoarthritis in dogs with bilateral medial patellar luxation and unilateral surgical repair. *Vet. Surg.* **1992**, *21*, 475–479. [CrossRef]
6. Miles, J.E.; Dickow, M.; Nielsen, D.H.; Jensen, B.R.; Kirpensteijn, J.; Svalastoga, E.L.; Eriksen, T. Five patellar proximodistal positioning indices compared in clinically normal Greenland sled dogs. *Vet. J.* **2012**, *193*, 529–534. [CrossRef]
7. Browne, C.; Hermida, J.C.; Bergula, A.; Colwell, C.W.; D'Lima, D.D. Patellofemoral forces after total knee arthroplasty: Effect of extensor moment arm. *Knee* **2005**, *12*, 81–88. [CrossRef] [PubMed]
8. Figgie, H.E.; Goldberg, V.M.; Heiple, K.G.; Moller, H.S.; Gordon, N.H. The influence of tibial-patellofemoral location on function of the knee in patients with the posterior stabilized condylar knee prothesis. *J. Bone Jt. Surg. Am.* **1986**, *68*, 1035–1040. [CrossRef]
9. Floren, M.; Davis, J.; Peterson, M.G.; Laskin, R.S. A mini-midvastus capsular approach with patellar displacement decreases the prevalence of patella baja. *J. Arthroplast.* **2007**, *22*, 51–57. [CrossRef]
10. Ghandi, R.; de Beer, J.; Leone, J.; Petruccelli, D.; Winemark, M.; Adili, A. Predictive risk factors for stiff knees in total knee arthroplasty. *J. Atrhroplasty* **2006**, *21*, 46–52.
11. Luyckx, T.; Didden, K.; Vandenneucker, H.; Labey, L.; Innocenti, B.; Bellemans, J. Is there a biomechanical explanation for anteror knee pain in patients with patella alta?: Influence of patellar height on patellofemoral contact force, contact area and contact pressure. *J. Bone Jt. Surg. Br.* **2009**, *91*, 344–350. [CrossRef] [PubMed]
12. Thaunat, M.; Erasmus, J.P. Recurrent patellar dislocation after medial patellofemoral ligament reconstruction. *Knee Surg. Sport. Traumatol. Arthrosc.* **2008**, *16*, 40–43. [CrossRef] [PubMed]
13. Aparicio, G.; Abril, J.C.; Calvo, E.; Alvarez, L. Radiologic study of patellar height in Osgood-Shaltter disease. *J. Pediatr. Orthop.* **1997**, *17*, 63–66. [CrossRef] [PubMed]
14. Hirano, A.; Fukubayashi, T.; Ishii, T.; Ochiai, N. Relationship between the patellar neight and the disorder of the knee extensor mechanism in immature athletes. *Pediatr. Orthop.* **2001**, *21*, 541–544. [CrossRef]
15. Visuri, T.; Pihlajamäki, H.K.; Mattila, V.M.; Kiuru, M. Elongated patellae at the final stage of Osgood-Shaltter disease: A radigraohic study. *Knee* **2007**, *14*, 198–203. [CrossRef] [PubMed]
16. Drexler, M.; Dwyer, T.; Marmor, M.; Sternheim, A.; Cameron, H.U.; Cameron, J.C. The treatment of acquired patella baja with proximalize the tibial tuberosity. *Knee Surg. Sports Traumatol. Arthrosc.* **2013**, *21*, 2578–2583. [CrossRef] [PubMed]
17. Paulos, L.E.; Rosenberg, T.D.; Drawbert, J.; Manning, J.; Abbott, P. Infrapatellar contracture syndrome: An unrecognize cause of knee stiffness with patella entrapment and patella infera. *Am. J. Sports Med.* **1987**, *15*, 331–341. [CrossRef] [PubMed]

18. Schiphof, D.; Middelkoop, M.; Klerk, B.M.; Oei, E.H.G.; Hofman, A.; Koes, B.W.; Weinans, H.; Zeinstra, S.M.A. Crepitus is a first indication of patellofemoral osteoarthritis (and not of tibiofemoral osteoarthiris). *Osteoa. Carti.* **2014**, *22*, 631–638. [CrossRef]
19. Bei, M.; Tian, F.; Liu, N.; Zheng, Z.; Cao, X.; Zhang, H.; Wang, Y.; Xiao, Y.; Dai, M.; Zhang, L. Anovel Rat Model of Patellofemoral Osteoarthritis Due to Patella Baja, or Low-Lying Patella. *Med. Sci. Monit.* **2019**, *13*, 2702–2717. [CrossRef]
20. Grelsamer, R.P.; Meadows, S. The modified Insall-Salvati ratio for assessment of patellar height. *Clin. Orthop. Relat. Res.* **1992**, *282*, 170–176. [CrossRef]
21. Johnson, A.L.; Probst, C.W.; DeCamp, C.E.; Rosenstein, D.S.; Hauptman, J.G.; Kern, T.L. Vertical position of the patella in the stifle joint of clinically normal large-breed dogs. *Am. J. Vet. Res.* **2002**, *63*, 42–46. [CrossRef] [PubMed]
22. Mostafa, A.A.; Griffon, D.J.; Thomas, W.M.; Constable, P.D. Proximodistal alignment of the canine patella: Radiographic evaluation and association with medial and lateral patellar luxation. *Vet. Surg.* **2008**, *37*, 201–2011. [CrossRef] [PubMed]
23. Vincenti, S.; Knell, S.; Pozzi, A. Surgical treatment of a proximal diaphyseal tibial deformity associated with partial caudal and cranial cruciate ligament deficiency and patella baja. *Schweiz. Arch. Tierheilk.* **2017**, *159*, 237–242. [CrossRef] [PubMed]
24. Knazovicky, D.; Ledecky, V.; Hluchy, M.; Durej, M. Use of modified Insall Salvati method for determination of vertical patellar position in dogs with and without cranial cruciate ligament rupture considering the morphology of the cranio-proximal tibia. *Acta. Vet. Brno* **2012**, *81*, 403–407. [CrossRef]
25. Lojszczyk, S.A.; Slimanowicz, P.; Komsta, R.; Osinski, Z. Determination of reference values and frequency of occurrence of patella alta in German shepherd dogs: A retrospective study. *Acta Vet. Scand.* **2017**, *59*, 36. [CrossRef] [PubMed]
26. Lorinson, K.; Winkler, M.; Lorinson, D.; Tichy, A. Radiographische Evaluierung der prä- und post-operativen Patellahöhe bei TPLO und TTA Patienten. *Wien. Tierarztl. Monat- Vet. Med. Austria* **2022**, *109*, Doc1. [CrossRef]
27. Ocal, M.K.; Seyrek-Intas, D.; Cagatay, S. Comparison of Insall-Salvati Index and its modification in normal dogs from four different body weight groups. *Vet. Comp. Othop. Traumatol.* **2020**, *33*, 110–115. [CrossRef] [PubMed]
28. Johnson, A.L.; Broaddus, K.D.; Hauptman, J.G.; Marsh, S.; Monsere, J.; Sepulveda, G. Vertical patellar position in large-breed dogs with clinically normal stifles and large-breed dogs with medial patellar luxation. *Vet. Surg.* **2006**, *35*, 78–81. [CrossRef] [PubMed]
29. Portner, O.; Pakzad, H. The evaluation of patellar height: A simple method. *J. Bone Jt. Surg. Am.* **2011**, *93*, 73–80. [CrossRef]
30. Murakami, S.; Shimada, M.; Harada, Y.; Hara, Y. Examination of the Proximodistal patellar position in small dogs in relation to anatomical features of the distal femur and medial patellar luxation. *PLoS ONE* **2021**, *5*, e0252531. [CrossRef]
31. Wangdee, C.; Theyse, L.F.H.; Hasewinkel, H.A.W. Proximo-distal patellar position in three small dogs breeds with medial patellar luxation. *Vet. Comp. Orthop. Traumatol.* **2015**, *28*, 270–273. [PubMed]
32. Bonadio, M.B.; Torres, J.A.P.; Filho, V.M.; Helito, C.P. Plateau-patella angle: An option for assessing patellar height on proximal tibia osteotomy. *Acta Orth. Bras.* **2016**, *24*, 127–130. [CrossRef] [PubMed]
33. Slocum, B.; Slocum, T.D. Tibial plateau leveling osteotomy for repair of cranial cruciate ligament rupture in the canine. *Vet. Clin. N. Am. Small Anin. Pract.* **1993**, *23*, 777–795. [CrossRef] [PubMed]
34. Reif, U.; Dejardin, L.M.; Probst, C.W.; DeCamp, C.E.; Flo, G.L.; Johnson, A.L. Influence of limb positioning and measurement method on the magnitude of the tibial plateau angle. *Vet. Surg.* **2004**, *33*, 368–375. [CrossRef] [PubMed]
35. Geier, M.C.; Frederick, S.W.; Cross, A.R. Evaluation of the risk of patella fracture as the result of decreasing tibial plateau angle following tibial plateau leveling osteotomy. *Vet. Surg.* **2021**, *50*, 984–989. [CrossRef] [PubMed]
36. Capkin, S.; Guler, S.; Sezgin, E. Comparison of five patellar height measurement methods in a Turkish adult cohort. *Ann. Med. Res.* **2020**, *27*, 1549–1553. [CrossRef]
37. Winkler, M. Radiologische Evaluierung der Patellaposition Anhand Spezifischer Indizes Bei Tibia Plateau Leveling Osteotomy und Tibial Tuberosity Advancement Bei Hunden. Master's Thesis, The University of Veterinary Medicine, Vienna, Austria, 2019.
38. Garnoeva, R.S. Evaluation of Proximodistal patellar alignment in small breed dogs with or without patellar luxation using the Insall-Salvati, Caton-Deschamps, and Blackburne-Peel indices. *Open Vet. J.* **2023**, *13*, 663–667. [CrossRef] [PubMed]
39. Feldmane, L.; Theyse, L.F.H. Proximodistal and caudocranial position of the insertion of the patellar ligament on the tibial tuberosity and patellar ligament length of normal stifle and stifle with grade II medial patellar luxation in small-breed dogs. *Vet. Surg.* **2021**, *50*, 1017–1022. [CrossRef] [PubMed]
40. Lorinson, K.; Kneissl, S.; Tichy, A.; Lorinson, D. Radiographic Measurement of the Patellar Height in Cats Using the Tibia Plateau-Patella Angle (TPPA). *Biomed. J. Sci. Tech. Res.* **2023**, *49*, 40929–40933.
41. De Carvalho, A.; Andersen, A.H.; Topp, S.; Jurik, A.G. A method for assessing the height of the patella. *Internat. Orthop.* **1985**, *9*, 195–197. [CrossRef]
42. Bound, N.; Zakai, D.; Butterworth, S.J.; Pead, M. Clinical features and radiographic evidence of limb deviation. *Vet. Comp. Orthop. Traumatol.* **2009**, *22*, 32–37. [PubMed]

Disclaimer/Publisher's Note: The statements, opinions and data contained in all publications are solely those of the individual author(s) and contributor(s) and not of MDPI and/or the editor(s). MDPI and/or the editor(s) disclaim responsibility for any injury to people or property resulting from any ideas, methods, instructions or products referred to in the content.

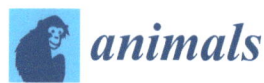

Article

Effects of the Direction of Two Kirschner Wires on Combined Tibial Plateau Leveling Osteotomy and Tibial Tuberosity Transposition in Miniature Breed Dogs: An Ex Vivo Study

Sanghyun Nam [†], Youngjin Jeon [†], Haebeom Lee and Jaemin Jeong *

Department of Veterinary Surgery, College of Veterinary Medicine, Chungnam National University, Daejeon 34134, Republic of Korea; nmdanny86@gmail.com (S.N.); orangee0115@gmail.com (Y.J.); seatiger76@cnu.ac.kr (H.L.)
* Correspondence: klmie800@cnu.ac.kr
[†] These authors contributed equally to this work.

Simple Summary: This study investigates how the direction of wire placement affects the stability of combined tibial plateau leveling osteotomy and tibial tuberosity transposition surgery in miniature-breed dogs suffering from two common stifle problems: a torn cruciate ligament and patella luxation. Using the bones from 21 small dogs, we tested pin placement in two directions: proximal (proximal osteotomized segment) and distal. This study also tested different wire thicknesses and the use of tension bands. The results showed that distal pin placement provided better stability in the 0.56 mm tension band group. This finding is important because it offers a solution for cases where there is not enough space to place pins in the proximal direction. In situations where there is inadequate space for proximal pin placement, distal pin placement can achieve similar stability. This research provides valuable insights that can lead to better surgical outcomes for small animal surgeons.

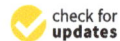

Citation: Nam, S.; Jeon, Y.; Lee, H.; Jeong, J. Effects of the Direction of Two Kirschner Wires on Combined Tibial Plateau Leveling Osteotomy and Tibial Tuberosity Transposition in Miniature Breed Dogs: An Ex Vivo Study. *Animals* **2024**, *14*, 2258. https://doi.org/10.3390/ani14152258

Academic Editors: L. Miguel Carreira and João Alves

Received: 8 July 2024
Revised: 24 July 2024
Accepted: 2 August 2024
Published: 3 August 2024

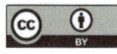

Copyright: © 2024 by the authors. Licensee MDPI, Basel, Switzerland. This article is an open access article distributed under the terms and conditions of the Creative Commons Attribution (CC BY) license (https:// creativecommons.org/licenses/by/ 4.0/).

Abstract: This study evaluates the impact of Kirschner wire (K-wire) insertion direction on the biomechanical properties of combined tibial plateau leveling osteotomy (TPLO) and tibial tuberosity transposition (TTT) procedures in small-breed dogs with cranial cruciate ligament rupture and medial patella luxation. Twenty-one cadaveric tibiae were divided into two groups; the specimens were divided into two groups; one underwent TPLO-TTT with a proximal pin placement (Group TTP) and the other received TPLO-TTT with a distal pin placement (Group TTD). For both pin placements, two additional subgroups were formed: one with a 0.56 mm tension band (Groups TTP0.56 and TTD0.56) and the other with a 0.76 mm tension band (Groups TTP0.76 and TTD0.76). The tensile force was applied, and failure load and mode were recorded. The distal pin direction in Group TTD0.56 exhibited a significantly higher mean failure load (380.1 N) compared to the proximal pin direction in Group TTP0.56 (302.2 N, $p = 0.028$). No significant differences were observed among the other groups. This study concludes that distal pin placement can provide similar or improved mechanical stability in cases with limited space for proximal pin placement during combined TPLO and TTT procedures.

Keywords: tibia plateau leveling osteotomy; tibial tuberosity transposition; Kirschner wire angle; tension band technique; dog

1. Introduction

Medial patellar luxation (MPL) and cranial cruciate ligament rupture (CCLR) represent predominant causes of hindlimb lameness within the canine population, exhibiting a particularly high prevalence among small-breed dogs [1–4]. According to previous studies, small breeds are significantly more susceptible to MPL, with a reported incidence rate up to 12 times higher than that observed in larger breeds [5,6]. Moreover, the occurrence of concurrent CCLR in patients diagnosed with MPL ranges from 22% to 44%, underscoring the clinical complexity and necessitating effective surgical interventions to restore limb function [7,8].

Surgical techniques for treating MPL commonly include a variety of techniques such as soft-tissue realignment, trochleoplasty, tibial tuberosity transposition (TTT), and distal femoral osteotomy [4]. The TTT method, specifically, addresses congenital or acquired malalignments of the quadriceps mechanism, a condition frequently accompanying MPL. A TTT is a common procedure performed in surgical correction of the medial patellar luxation in dogs [2,4]. This technique involves the osteotomy and subsequent repositioning of a tibia tuberosity segment to counteract the luxation direction, secured in its new location with surgical implants [1,3,4,9]. In cases of CCLR, procedures like tibia plateau leveling osteotomy (TPLO), CORA-based leveling osteotomy (CBLO), and tibia tuberosity advancement (TTA) are integrated to effectively address joint instability [10,11].

Recent studies have reported several methods that address concurrent MPL and CCLR within a single session. These methods, including modified TPLO (mTPLO), tibia tuberosity transposition advancement (TTTA), and combined TPLO with TTT, aim to address quadriceps malalignment and stabilize the CCL-deficient stifle joints [10–14]. Various techniques have been explored to improve the mechanical stability and clinical outcomes of these procedures. Although previous ex vivo studies evaluating combined TPLO-TTT report that TPLO-TTT has weaker mechanical stability compared to TTT or TPLO alone [15], it has been shown to provide relatively good short- to long-term outcomes in retrospective clinical studies [11,16,17].

However, performing combined TPLO-TTT in miniature-breed dogs can be challenging in surgical precision, particularly with the insertion of Kirschner wire (K-wire) for TTT fixation. This difficulty mainly arises from the impingement of pins on TPLO screws in the rotated proximal tibial plateau segment. Alternatively, K-wires can be inserted in the distal direction instead of the proximal direction into the proximal tibial plateau segment. However, there is a lack of studies on how the biomechanical properties of TTT fixation in TPLO-TTT change when the insertion direction of these K-wires is altered.

Therefore, the purpose of this study is to analyze the biomechanical effects of the Kirschner wire insertion angle (KWIA), in the combined TPLO-TTT technique in 2–5 kg miniature-breed dogs. Our hypothesis was that there would be no difference in load at failure or mode of failure between the direction of the K-wire, regardless of whether a tension band (TB) was applied or the size of the TB wire if applied.

2. Materials and Methods

2.1. Specimens and Preparation

Twenty-one donated miniature-breed cadavers weighing between 2 and 5 kg, euthanatized for reasons unrelated to this study, were included in the ex vivo study. The ethics approval for the cadaveric study protocol was not required by the Institutional Animal Care and Use Committee of Chungnam National University. Cadavers were preserved at −20 °C and thawed to room temperature (21 °C) prior to experimentation. Comprehensive craniocaudal and mediolateral radiographic of each tibia were performed with a 25 mm radiographic marker for precise measurement. The specimens were then divided into six groups based on the specific surgical technique applied and the size of the tension band (TB). Each group included 6 tibiae, representing either the left or right hindlimb from one individual dog.

The groups were divided as follows: Group TTP: TPLO + TTT with the proximal insertion of two K-wires, no tension band; Group TTD: TPLO + TTT with the distal insertion of two K-wires, no tension band; Group TTP0.56: TPLO + TTT with the proximal insertion of two K-wires and a 0.56 mm tension band; Group TTD0.56: TPLO + TTT with the distal insertion of two K-wires and a 0.56 mm tension band; Group TTP0.76: TPLO + TTT with the proximal insertion of two K-wires and a 0.76 mm tension band; and Group TTD0.76: TPLO + TTT with the distal insertion of two K-wires and a 0.76 mm tension band.

A coin flip method was used to assign the left or right hindlimb of each group. For example, if the left hindlimb was assigned to the TTP group, the right hindlimb from the same dog was assigned to the TTD group, ensuring that each dog provided paired samples for comparison. The two K-wires were inserted parallel to each other at the same level. This process was similarly applied to the TTP0.56 group (TTP + 0.56 mm TB) and the TTD0.56 group (TTD + 0.56 mm tension band wire), as well as the TTP0.76 group (TTP + 0.76 mm tension band wire) and the TTD0.76 group (TTD + 0.76 mm tension band wire) (Figure 1). The remaining three pairs of the hindlimb were included as a control group, which only underwent TPLO.

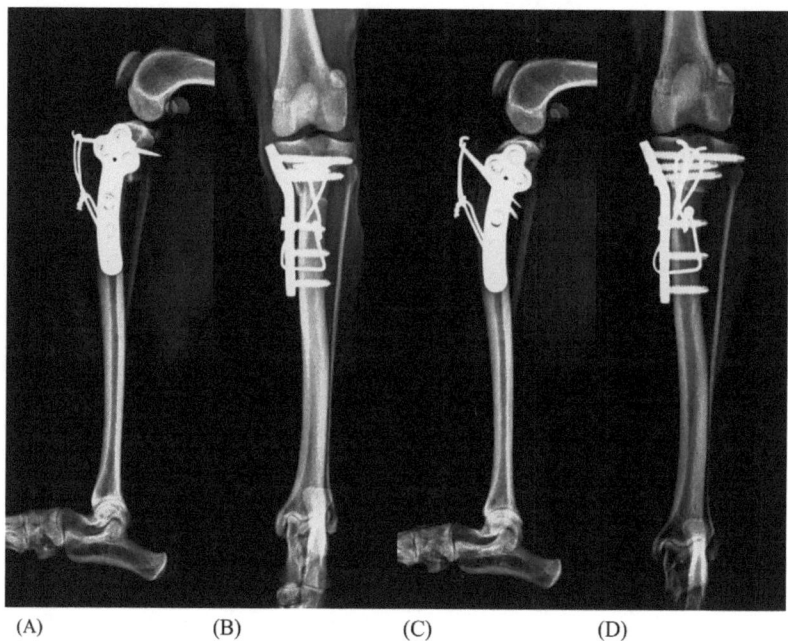

(A)   (B)   (C)   (D)

Figure 1. Craniocaudal and mediolateral radiographs of the TTP0.76 (**A**,**B**) and TTD0.76 (**C**,**D**) groups. The tension band was applied in a figure-eight pattern, and the pins were 1.0 mm and 0.8 mm.

2.2. Surgical Techniques

Preoperative TPLO planning was performed using digital software vPOP (vPOP Pro version 2.9.6, VetSOS Education Ltd., Shrewsbury, UK). TPLO and TTT were conducted on all 36 tibiae following established protocols from a previous study [9,18]. A 12 mm crescentic saw blade was used for the osteotomy, placing the intercondylar eminence as the central point. Temporary fixation was performed with a 1.0 K-wire after rotation of the tibial plateau segment and achieving a tibial plateau angle (TPA) of 6°, and a 2.0 mm TPLO bone plate (Able Inc., Jeonju, Republic of Korea) was used for osteotomy stabilization [19]. Following plate application, TTT was performed using an oscillating saw (DePuy Synthes Vet, Oberdorf, Switzerland) to ensure a linear osteotomy and to preserve the craniodistal periosteal attachment. The osteotomized segment was laterally translated into a distance of one-third of the tibia tuberosity's width. K-wires were inserted at the proximal insertion point of the patellar ligament to secure the segment, passing through and emerging from the opposite tibial cortex. TB was applied as a single twist to the TTP-0.56, TTD-0.56, TTP-0.76, and TTD-0.76 groups.

2.3. Radiographic Measurements

Orthogonal radiographs of each pair of tibiae were obtained to assess the pin insertion angle and postoperative TPA using commercially available radiographic software (Zetta PACS Viewer 2001, Taeyoung Soft Co., Ltd., Gwacheon, Republic of Korea). K-wire insertion angles were determined on lateral radiographs by measuring the angle between the osteotomy line and the inserted K-wire, as described in a previous study (Figure 2) [20]. The two K-wires were assigned as P1 and P2, and the data were obtained as the mean standard deviation of the K-wire angle by calculating [P1 + P2]/2.

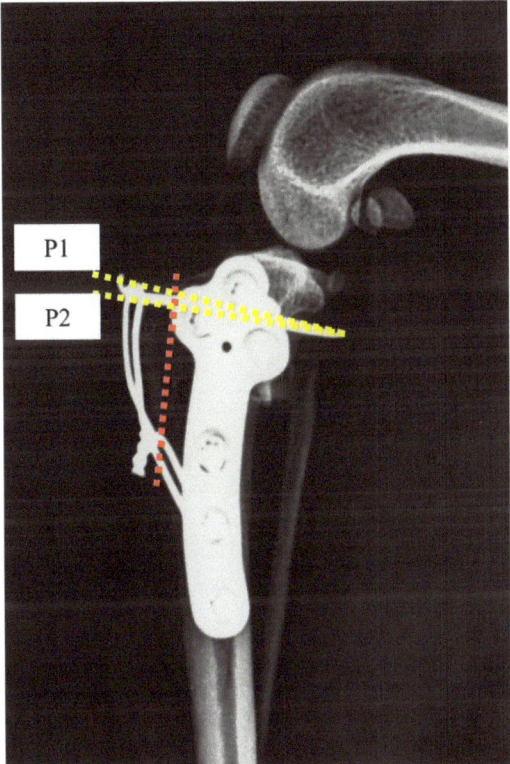

Figure 2. K-wire insertion angle (KWIA) was measured using Zetta PACS (Taeyoung Soft Co., Ltd., Gwacheon, Republic of Korea). The angle formed by the K-wire and the osteotomy line (red dotted line) was measured. The two K-wires were assigned as P1 and P2 (yellow dotted line), and the data were obtained as the mean standard deviation of the K-wire angle by calculating [P1 + P2]/2.

2.4. Mechanical Testing

Specimens were mounted in a 35 mm internal diameter stainless steel pipe using methyl methacrylate resin (Trayplast, Vertex, Soesterberg, The Netherlands) and then attached to a loading cell within a custom-designed jig. The tibiae were then secured to the load cell using a custom-designed jig. The patellar tendon was secured to the actuator using a custom-made clamp (Figure 3). The jig was configured to hold the tibia and patellar ligament at 135 degrees to mimic the midstance angle of the stifle of dogs [21]. A testing machine (WL2100C, WITHLAB Co., Ltd., Gunpo, Republic of Korea) was used to perform vertical distraction at a displacement rate of 20 mm/min until failure of the tibia construct was observed. The load at failure (Newtons) and the mode of failure were recorded for each specimen. All testing was video-recorded (iPhone 14, Apple Inc., Cupertino, CA, USA) with the load display and tibias on the same screen (Figure 3).

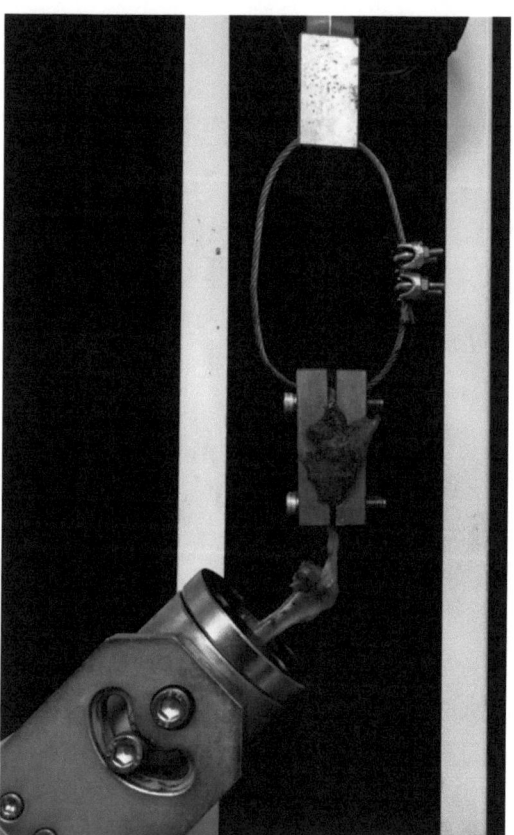

Figure 3. Biomechanical testing setup. Specimens were mounted using methyl methacrylate resin (Trayplast, Vertex, Soesterberg, The Netherlands) in a stainless steel pipe with an inner diameter of 35 mm. The specimens were secured to the loading cell, and the patellar tendon was fixed at an angle of 135° in a custom-designed clamp.

2.5. Statistical Analysis

Based on the results of a previous study [20], a prospective power analysis was conducted using statistical software (G*Power V3.1.9.2x Dusseldorf, Germany), and it was determined that a sample size of 6 constructs (n = 6 tibia/group) would have alpha = 0.05, power = 0.8 and an estimated effect size (ES, d = 1.4790362). Statistical analysis was performed using commercially available software (IBM SPSS Statistics 24.0, IBM Corp., Chicago, IL, USA). Data were nonparametrically distributed, and postoperative K-wire angle and load at failure were evaluated between the groups using the Wilcoxon test and Kruskal–Wallis test. The Mann–Whitney U test was used for post hoc analysis. Statistical significance was set at a value of $p < 0.05$.

3. Results

All cadavers met the criteria with a total of 36 stifles and were skeletally mature. The median body weight was 3.6 kg (range: 2–5 kg), and there were 13 intact females, 2 spayed females, and 3 intact males. The most dominant breed was Poodle (n = 9), followed by

Maltese ($n = 4$), Bichon ($n = 2$), Chihuahua ($n = 1$), and Pomeranian ($n = 1$). Descriptive data, including body weight, failure modes, preoperative tibial plateau angle, postoperative plateau angle, and the K-wire insertion number, are described in Table 1. Biomechanical test results and KWIA are described in Table 2.

Table 1. Comparison of body weight, tibial plateau angle (TPA), pin insertion number, and failure mode.

	Body Weight (Kg)	Preoperative TPA	Postoperative TPA	Pin Insertion Number	Failure Mode
Group 1 TTP	3.62 ± 0.38	28.90 ± 4.35°	6.33 ± 2.34°	0 ($n = 1$), 1 ($n = 2$), 2 ($n = 2$), 3 ($n = 1$)	Avulsion ($n = 6$)
Group 2 TTD	3.62 ± 0.38	28.67 ± 3.37°	5.33 ± 1.51°	0 ($n = 5$), 1 ($n = 1$)	Avulsion ($n = 6$)
Group 3 TTP0.56	3.92 ± 0.71	30.70 ± 3.16°	6.33 ± 2.73°	0 ($n = 1$), 1 ($n = 2$), 2 ($n = 3$)	Avulsion ($n = 3$), Fracture ($n = 3$)
Group 4 TTD0.56	3.92 ± 0.71	30.13 ± 3.07°	5.83 ± 2.99°	0 ($n = 5$), 1 ($n = 1$)	Tendon rupture ($n = 2$), Avulsion ($n = 3$), Fracture ($n = 1$)
Group 5 TTP0.76	3.34 ± 0.37	30.63 ± 3.13°	6.67 ± 2.07°	1 ($n = 2$), 2 ($n = 1$), 3 ($n = 2$)	Fracture ($n = 6$)
Group 6 TTD0.76	3.34 ± 0.37	30.20 ± 3.12°	6.33 ± 1.51°	0 ($n = 6$)	Fracture ($n = 6$)
Control TPLO	3.45 ± 0.45	25.47 ± 6.45°	7.17 ± 1.33°		Fracture ($n = 6$)

TTP, TPLO-TTT with proximal pin; TTD, TPLO-TTT with distal pin; TTP0.56, TPLO-TTT with proximal pin and 0.56 tension band; TTD0.56, TPLO-TTT with distal pin and 0.56 tension band; TTP0.76, TPLO-TTT with proximal pin and 0.76 tension band; TTD0.76, TPLO-TTT with distal pin and 0.76 tension band.

Table 2. Comparison of load at failure, yield force, periosteal bridge failure, and K-wire insertion angle by group.

	Group 1 TTP	Group 2 TTD	Group 3 TTP0.56	Group 4 TTD0.56	Group 5 TTP0.76	Group 6 TTD0.76	TPLO Control
Load at failure (N)	124.23 ±102.62	142.54 ±97.01	302.24 ±52.92 [a]	380.15 ±58.30 [a]	255.20 ±44.50	241.07 ±66.41	242.38 ±31.98
Yield force (N)	119.36 ±107.05	132.61 ±105.61	229.48 ±126.57	282.53 ±100.06	210.42 ±32.22	172.24 ±32.55	214.23 ±69.95
Periosteal bridge failure	6/6	6/6	3/6	5/6	N/A	N/A	N/A
K-wire insertion angle (°)	72.58 ±3.71 [b]	48.52 ±9.14 [b]	73.81 ±3.87 [a]	46.94 ±11.87 [a]	76.26 ±8.16 [c]	47.48 ±2.54 [c]	N/A

TTP, TPLO-TTT with proximal pin; TTD, TPLO-TTT with distal pin; TTP0.56, TPLO-TTT with proximal pin and 0.56 tension band; TTD0.56, TPLO-TTT with distal pin and 0.56 tension band; TTP0.76, TPLO-TTT with proximal pin and 0.76 tension band; TTD0.76, TPLO-TTT with distal pin and 0.76 tension band; [a] p-value between Group 3 and 4 showed a significant difference, [b] p-value between Group 1 and 2 showed a significant difference, [c] p-value between Group 5 and 6 showed a significant difference; $p < 0.05$ was set as significant difference.

In the comparison of the proximal pin load at failure, TTP0.56 exhibited significantly greater strength compared to TTP ($p = 0.016$). Similarly, TTP0.76 demonstrated significantly greater strength than TTP ($p = 0.037$). However, the difference between TTP0.56 and TTP0.76 was not statistically significant, although it was close to significance ($p = 0.078$). For the distal pin load at failure, TTD0.56 showed significantly greater strength compared to TTD ($p = 0.004$). Additionally, TTD0.56 demonstrated significantly greater strength than TTD0.76 ($p = 0.01$). However, the difference between TTD and TTD0.76 was not significant ($p = 0.109$).

In the TTP and TTD groups, in which a TB was not applied, tibial tuberosity avulsion failure was observed (Figure 4). However, fractures were observed in some of the 0.56 tension band (TB) groups (TTP0.56 and TTD0.56) and all the 0.76 tension band (TB) groups (TTP0.76 and TTD0.76) as failure modes. The fracture occurred at the level where the tibia was embedded in the resin, precisely at the most superficial interface between the two materials. The number of fractures observed per group is specified in Table 1. In specimens that had more than one trial of proximal K-wire insertion, pin bending (Figure 5A) and locking screw damage was observed (Figure 5B). In the proximal pin groups (TTP, TTP0.56, and TTP0.76), damaged locking screws were found in proximal locking screws, whereas in the distal pin groups (TTD, TTD0.56, and TTD0.76), no screw damage was observed.

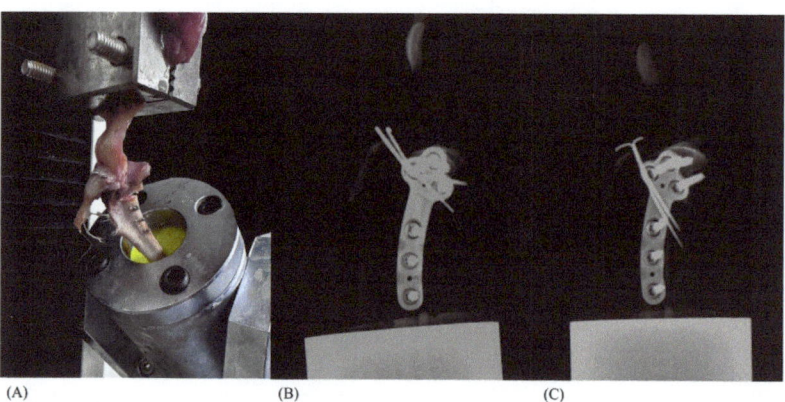

Figure 4. Photograph of tibial tuberosity avulsion failure mode (**A**) and mediolateral radiograph of TTP (**B**) and TTD (**C**). Distal periosteum breakage is observed, along with bending of both the proximal pin and distal K-wires.

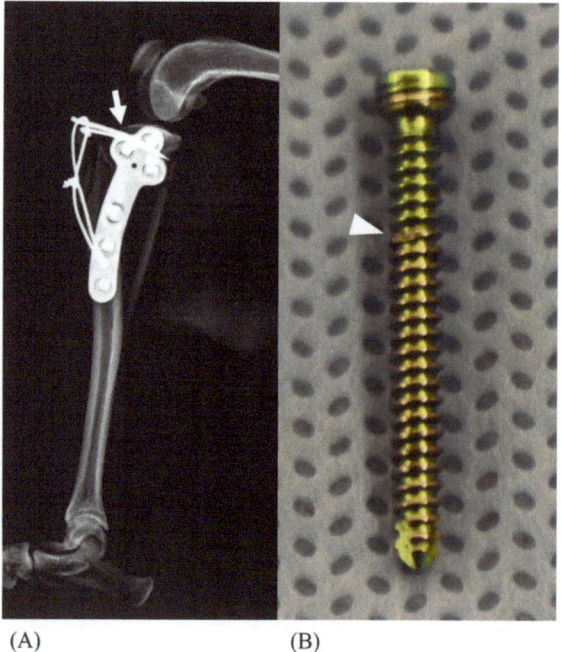

Figure 5. Mediolateral radiograph of the proximal pin group (**A**). During pin insertion, the pin bends due to the limited space caused by the proximal tibial plateau segment locking screw (arrow). The photograph of the damaged proximal locking screw due to K-wire insertion (**B**).

The comparison of KWIA between the proximal pin groups and the distal pin groups was significant ($p = 0.000$). The TTP and TTD groups showed a significant difference ($p = 0.028$), as did the TTP0.56 and TTD0.56 groups ($p = 0.028$); similarly, the TTP0.76 and TTD0.76 groups showed a significant difference ($p = 0.028$).

4. Discussion

This study evaluated the biomechanical properties of combined TTT and TPLO depending on the direction of the Kirschner wire insertion angle and the application of the tension band. Our hypothesis posited that there would be no significant difference in the biomechanical integrity, load at failure, or mode of failure between proximal pin placement and distal pin placement. This hypothesis was partially accepted, as groups TTP, TTD, TTP0.76, and TTD0.76 showed no difference in load at failure and mode of failure. However, between the TTP0.56 and TTD0.56 groups, a significant difference was observed in the load at failure, with the distal pin group showing higher mechanical strength.

According to previous studies [20,22–24], inserting the pin in a caudodistal or transverse direction is known to provide better counteraction against the patellar tendon force during TTT surgery. Additionally, the AO principle for TB to manage fractures recommends the placement of two parallel pins across and perpendicular to the fracture plane [25]. However, in the current study, inserting the K-wire perpendicular to the TTT osteotomy line and into the proximal tibial plateau segment to stabilize the osteotomized tuberosity segment posed a challenge. This difficulty arose because of the conflict between the pins and the proximal locking screw due to the narrow space in the proximal tibial plateau segment, especially in miniature breed dogs. Therefore, in the proximal pin groups, the pin was inserted at a mean angle of 74.23 degrees to the osteotomy line.

Inserting the K-wire into the proximal tibial plateau segment caused resistance with the proximal locking screw, resulting in multiple insertion attempts in groups TTP, TTP0.56, and TTP0.76. Although the wire eventually flexed slightly and passed through, this process caused damage to the threads of the locking screw (Figure 5A). Additionally, these attempts increased the space where the K-wire passed through, which can lead to implant loosening in a clinical setting.

The failure mode observed in groups TTP, TTD, TTP0.56, and TTD0.56 was similar to that reported in studies on TPLO-TTT with or without a tension band, involving distal tibial crest displacement and rupture of the patellar ligament [15,26]. However, fracture occurred at the diaphysis of the tibia in four specimens, with three in TTP0.56 and one in TTD0.56 groups. This failure mode was consistent with observations from a previous TTT study [23]. The occurrence of such failures may be attributed to histological damage during freeze–thaw process of the specimens or differences in bone quality between specimens. However, if such failures were to occur in a clinical setting, they could have catastrophic consequences. Therefore, further research is necessary to assess the stress distribution in TPLO-TTT constructs with and without a tension band.

One of the interesting findings in the current study was that the failure mode in the TTP0.76 and TTD0.76 groups involved fractures at the junction between the tibia and the resin. In contrast to the 0.56TB group, where two out of the four fractured specimens experienced distal periosteum breakage, the specimens in the 0.76TB group all had intact distal periosteum. Although the actual mechanical test results showed that the 0.56TB specimens performed better than the 0.76TB specimens, the test results and failure modes may be attributed to the stress shielding effect [27,28] or stress concentration occurring at the junction where the tibia and cement, which have different material properties [29–31]. This result presents a clinical dilemma when choosing the appropriate tension band size in practice. Despite the expectation that the thicker 0.76TB would withstand higher mechanical loads, tibia diaphyseal fractures occurred at lower loads compared to the avulsion fractures observed in the 0.56TB group. These findings are in contradiction with the results reported by Neat and colleagues, which showed that larger TB sizes generally provide higher mechanical strength in an olecranon osteotomy model [32]. Therefore, further research is needed to determine the appropriate TB size based on bone size or patient weight. Additionally, it should be noted that this study used only one twist knot for securing the tension band wire due to the small bone size. According to a previous study, placing two knots results in more rigid fixation to the construct compared to a single knot [33]. One twist knot may not provide uniform tension across the entire wire, especially in larger bones, potentially resulting in less effective tightening compared to using two twist knots.

According to a previous study, the approximate quadriceps muscle force during walking for dogs in the weight range of the current study is 33.68 N [34]. All groups in our experiment, regardless of TB application and pin direction, exhibited forces higher than this value. However, in the TTP and TTD groups in which only pins were applied, the load at failure ranged from 39.37 N to 301.11 N, suggesting a potential risk of construct failure under conditions of higher forces such as those encountered during trotting. In contrast, the 0.56 TB groups showed a load at failure ranging from 227.56 N to 480.03 N, and the 0.76 TB groups exhibited a load at failure ranging from 164.16 N to 349.46 N. These results suggest significantly improved mechanical stability when a TB is applied. Therefore, it is cautiously recommended to apply TBs during TPLO-TTT in a clinical setting.

Our study has limitations, and caution is required for direct clinical application. First, since our study was designed ex vivo, with muscles and ligaments removed from the tibia except for the quadriceps muscle and patellar tendon. Therefore, the results may not fully replicate the actual weight-bearing situation. In clinical settings, the soft tissue and callus formation around the proximal tibia may provide additional resistance. Secondly, since all surgical procedures were performed by a single surgeon, outcomes related to experience may vary, including a potential bias where the 0.56 mm wire might have been tightened more stably due to ease of manipulation compared to the thicker 0.76 mm wire when applying the TB. Thirdly, we could not clarify the mechanism of fracture observed in the 0.76 TB groups. Although the results showed no significant differences based on pin direction in the 0.76 TB groups, further study is necessary, as different outcomes may arise when conducting the procedure on larger bone specimens.

5. Conclusions

In conclusion, our study primarily aimed to analyze the biomechanical effects of the Kirschner wire insertion angle in the combined TPLO-TTT technique for 2–5 kg miniature-breed dogs. Our finding suggests that, in general, the direction of the K-wire does not significantly affect stability, except when using a 0.56 mm tension band. When a 2.0 mm TPLO plate and a 0.56 TB are used for the combined TPLO and TTT, inserting the K-wire distally may be considered if proximal pin insertion is challenging due to the proximal locking screw. Furthermore, significant differences were observed when a TB was not applied during TPLO-TTT compared to the TB-applied group. Therefore, in clinical settings, the application of TBs is recommended during TPLO-TTT to avoid the risk of construct failure.

Author Contributions: Conceptualization, H.L. and S.N.; methodology S.N.; software, S.N. and Y.J.; validation, H.L. and J.J.; formal analysis, S.N and J.J.; investigation, S.N.; resources, S.N. and Y.J.; data curation, S.N.; writing—original draft preparation, S.N. and Y.J.; writing—review and editing, H.L., J.J. and Y.J.; visualization, S.N.; supervision, H.L. and J.J.; project administration, H.L. and J.J. All authors have read and agreed to the published version of the manuscript.

Funding: This work was supported by the Seoul Business Agency through the Seoul R&BD Program (BT230135)—Bio·Medicine Technology Commercialization, funded by Seoul City.

Institutional Review Board Statement: Ethical approval for the cadaveric study protocol was not required by the Institutional Animal Care and Use Committee of Chungnam National University, as the cadavers were donated by their owners, and euthanasia was unrelated to this study.

Informed Consent Statement: Informed consent was obtained from all the subjects involved in the study.

Data Availability Statement: The original data used in this study are included in the article; further inquiries can be directed to the corresponding author.

Acknowledgments: The authors thank ABLE Inc. for donating the TPLO implants used in this study.

Conflicts of Interest: The authors declare no conflicts of interest.

References

1. Arthurs, G.I.; Langley-Hobbs, S.J. Complications associated with corrective surgery for patellar luxation in 109 dogs. *Vet. Surg.* **2006**, *35*, 559–566. [CrossRef] [PubMed]
2. Kowaleski, M.P.; Boudrieau, R.J.; Pozzi, A.; Tobias, K.M.; Johnston, S.A. Stifle joint. In *Veterinary Surgery: Small Animal*, 2nd ed.; Johnston, S.A., Tobias, K.M., Eds.; Elsevier: St. Louis, MI, USA, 2017; Volume 1, pp. 1071–1168.
3. LaFond, E.; Breur, G.J.; Austin, C.C. Breed susceptibility for developmental orthopedic diseases in dogs. *J. Am. Anim. Hosp. Assoc.* **2002**, *38*, 467–477. [CrossRef] [PubMed]
4. Perry, K.L.; Dejardin, L.M. Canine medial patellar luxation. *J. Small Anim. Pract.* **2021**, *62*, 315–335. [CrossRef] [PubMed]
5. Alam, M.; Lee, J.; Kang, H.; Kim, I.; Park, S.; Lee, K.; Kim, N. Frequency and distribution of patellar luxation in dogs. *Vet. Comp. Orthop. Traumatol.* **2007**, *20*, 59–64. [CrossRef] [PubMed]
6. Priester, W.A. Sex, size, and breed as risk factors in canine patellar dislocation. *J. Am. Vet. Med. Assoc.* **1972**, *160*, 740–742. [PubMed]
7. Campbell, C.A.; Horstman, C.L.; Mason, D.R.; Evans, R.B. Severity of patellar luxation and frequency of concomitant cranial cruciate ligament rupture in dogs: 162 cases (2004–2007). *J. Am. Vet. Med. Assoc.* **2010**, *236*, 887–891. [CrossRef] [PubMed]
8. Candela Andrade, M.; Slunsky, P.; Klass, L.G.; Brunnberg, L. Risk factors and long-term surgical outcome of patellar luxation and concomitant cranial cruciate ligament rupture in small breed dogs. *Vet. Med.* **2020**, *65*, 159–167. [CrossRef]
9. Singleton, W. The diagnosis and surgical treatment of some abnormal stifle conditions in the dog. *Vet. Rec.* **1957**, *69*, 1387–1394.
10. Clough, W.T.; Dycus, D.L.; Barnhart, M.D.; Hulse, D.A.; Litsky, A.S. Combined center of rotation of angulation-based leveling osteotomy and tibial tuberosity transposition: An ex vivo mechanical study. *Vet. Surg.* **2022**, *51*, 489–496. [CrossRef]
11. Leonard, K.C.; Kowaleski, M.P.; Saunders, W.B.; McCarthy, R.J.; Boudrieau, R.J. Combined tibial plateau levelling osteotomy and tibial tuberosity transposition for treatment of cranial cruciate ligament insufficiency with concomitant medial patellar luxation. *Vet. Comp. Orthop. Traumatol.* **2016**, *29*, 536–540. [CrossRef]
12. Yeadon, R.; Fitzpatrick, N.; Kowaleski, M. Tibial tuberosity transposition-advancement for treatment of medial patellar luxation and concomitant cranial cruciate ligament disease in the dog. *Vet. Comp. Orthop. Traumatol.* **2011**, *24*, 18–26. [CrossRef] [PubMed]
13. Jeong, E.; Jeon, Y.; Kim, T.; Lee, D.; Roh, Y. Assessing the Effectiveness of Modified Tibial Plateau Leveling Osteotomy Plates for Treating Cranial Cruciate Ligament Rupture and Medial Patellar Luxation in Small-Breed Dogs. *Animals* **2024**, *14*, 1937. [CrossRef] [PubMed]
14. Dallago, M.; Baroncelli, A.B.; Hudson, C.; Peirone, B.; De Bakker, E.; Piras, L.A. Effect of Plate Type on Tibial Plateau Levelling and Medialization Osteotomy for Treatment of Cranial Cruciate Ligament Rupture and Concomitant Medial Patellar Luxation in Small Breed Dogs: An In Vitro Study. *Vet. Comp. Orthop. Traumatol.* **2023**, *36*, 212–217. [CrossRef] [PubMed]
15. Birks, R.R.; Kowaleski, M.P. Combined Tibial Plateau Levelling Osteotomy and Tibial Tuberosity Transposition: An Ex Vivo Mechanical Study. *Vet. Comp. Orthop. Traumatol.* **2018**, *31*, 124–130. [CrossRef]
16. Redolfi, G.; Grand, J.G. Complications and Long-Term Outcomes after Combined Tibial Plateau Leveling Osteotomy and Tibial Tuberosity Transposition for Treatment of Concurrent Cranial Cruciate Ligament Rupture and Grade III or IV Medial Patellar Luxation. *Vet. Comp. Orthop. Traumatol.* **2024**, *37*, 43–49. [CrossRef] [PubMed]
17. Cook, J.L.; Evans, R.; Conzemius, M.G.; Lascelles, B.D.X.; McIlwraith, C.W.; Pozzi, A.; Clegg, P.; Innes, J.; Schulz, K.; Houlton, J. Proposed definitions and criteria for reporting time frame, outcome, and complications for clinical orthopedic studies in veterinary medicine. *Vet. Surg.* **2010**, *39*, 905–908. [CrossRef] [PubMed]
18. Slocum, B.; Slocum, T.D. Tibial plateau leveling osteotomy for repair of cranial cruciate ligament rupture in the canine. *Vet. Clin. N. Am. Small Anim. Pract.* **1993**, *23*, 777–795. [CrossRef]
19. Windolf, M.; Leitner, M.; Schwieger, K.; Pearce, S.G.; Zeiter, S.; Schneider, E.; Johnson, K.A. Accuracy of fragment positioning after TPLO and effect on biomechanical stability. *Vet. Surg.* **2008**, *37*, 366–373. [CrossRef]
20. Hawbecker, T.J.; Duffy, D.J.; Chang, Y.J.; Moore, G.E. Influence of Kirschner-Wire Insertion Angle on Construct Biomechanics following Tibial Tuberosity Osteotomy Fixation in Dogs. *Vet. Comp. Orthop. Traumatol.* **2023**, *36*, 75–81. [CrossRef]
21. Dismukes, D.I.; Tomlinson, J.L.; Fox, D.B.; Cook, J.L.; Song, K.J.E. Radiographic measurement of the proximal and distal mechanical joint angles in the canine tibia. *Vet. Surg.* **2007**, *36*, 699–704. [CrossRef]
22. Cashmore, R.G.; Havlicek, M.; Perkins, N.R.; James, D.R.; Fearnside, S.M.; Marchevsky, A.M.; Black, A.P. Major complications and risk factors associated with surgical correction of congenital medial patellar luxation in 124 dogs. *Vet. Comp. Orthop. Traumatol.* **2014**, *27*, 263–270. [CrossRef] [PubMed]
23. Natsios, P.; Capaul, R.; Kopf, N.; Pozzi, A.; Tinga, S.; Park, B. Biomechanical evaluation of a fixation technique with a modified hemicerclage for tibial tuberosity transposition: An ex vivo cadaveric study. *Front. Vet. Sci.* **2024**, *11*, 1375380. [CrossRef] [PubMed]

24. Zide, A.N.; Jones, S.C.; Litsky, A.S.; Kieves, N.R. A Cadaveric Evaluation of Pin and Tension Band Configuration Strength for Tibial Tuberosity Osteotomy Fixation. *Vet. Comp. Orthop. Traumatol.* **2020**, *33*, 9–14. [CrossRef] [PubMed]
25. Roe, S.C. External fixators, pins, nails, and wires. In *AO Principles of Fracture Management in the Dog and Cat*; Johnson, A.L., Houlton, J.E., Vannini, R., Eds.; AO Pub.: Dübendorf, Switerland, 2005; pp. 53–71.
26. Newman, M.; Bertollo, N.; Walsh, W.; Voss, K. Tibial tuberosity transposition-advancement for lateralization of the tibial tuberosity: An ex vivo canine study. *Vet. Comp. Orthop. Traumatol.* **2014**, *27*, 271–276. [CrossRef] [PubMed]
27. Samiezadeh, S.; Avval, P.T.; Fawaz, Z.; Bougherara, H. On optimization of a composite bone plate using the selective stress shielding approach. *J. Mech. Behav. Biomed. Mater.* **2015**, *42*, 138–153. [CrossRef] [PubMed]
28. Wolff, J. *The Law of Bone Remodelling*, 1st ed.; Springer: Berlin/Heidelberg, Germnay, 1986.
29. Lauke, B. Stress concentration along curved interfaces as basis for adhesion tests. *Compos. Interfaces* **2007**, *14*, 307–320. [CrossRef]
30. Lipner, J.; Liu, W.; Liu, Y.; Boyle, J.; Genin, G.; Xia, Y.; Thomopoulos, S. The mechanics of PLGA nanofiber scaffolds with biomimetic gradients in mineral for tendon-to-bone repair. *J. Mech. Behav. Biomed. Mater.* **2014**, *40*, 59–68. [CrossRef] [PubMed]
31. Neves, A.d.A.; Coutinho, E.; Cardoso, M.V.; Jaecques, S.; Lambrechts, P.; Vander Sloten, J.; Van Oosterwyck, H.; Van Meerbeek, B. Influence of notch geometry and interface on stress concentration and distribution in micro-tensile bond strength specimens. *J. Dent.* **2008**, *36*, 808–815. [CrossRef]
32. Neat, B.C.; Kowaleski, M.P.; Litsky, A.S.; Boudrieau, R.J. Mechanical evaluation of pin and tension-band wire factors in an olecranon osteotomy model. *Vet. Surg.* **2006**, *35*, 398–405. [CrossRef]
33. Hak, D.J.; Golladay, G.J. Olecranon fractures: Treatment options. *J. Am. Acad. Orthop. Surg.* **2000**, *8*, 266–275. [CrossRef]
34. Shahar, R.; Banks-Sills, L. Biomechanical analysis of the canine hind limb: Calculation of forces during three-legged stance. *Vet. J.* **2002**, *163*, 240–250. [CrossRef] [PubMed]

Disclaimer/Publisher's Note: The statements, opinions and data contained in all publications are solely those of the individual author(s) and contributor(s) and not of MDPI and/or the editor(s). MDPI and/or the editor(s) disclaim responsibility for any injury to people or property resulting from any ideas, methods, instructions or products referred to in the content.

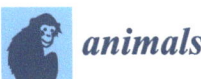

Case Report

Application of Hybrid External Skeletal Fixation with Bone Tissue Engineering Techniques for Comminuted Fracture of the Proximal Radius in a Dog

Minji Bae [1], Byung-Jae Kang [2] and Junhyung Kim [1,*]

1. Department of Veterinary Medicine, College of Veterinary Medicine and Institute of Veterinary Science, Kangwon National University, Chuncheon 24341, Republic of Korea; mangdi1224@kangwon.ac.kr
2. Department of Veterinary Clinical Sciences, College of Veterinary Medicine and Research Institute for Veterinary Science, Seoul National University, Seoul 08826, Republic of Korea; bjkang81@snu.ac.kr
* Correspondence: vetsurgeon@kangwon.ac.kr; Tel.: +82-33-250-8681

Simple Summary: This case report follows the recovery of a seven-month-old Pomeranian who had a serious fracture in its forelimb. The patient needed two surgeries to fix the fracture and help the bone heal using advanced methods. First, an external frame was used to keep the bone in place, along with a special material to help the bone grow. Although the bone initially healed well, problems with the frame caused the need for a second surgery. In the second surgery, a plate was added to support the bone, and a new healing material was used. After almost five years, the patient had less movement in the injured leg but did not seem to be in pain. X-rays showed only small changes in the joints, and although CT scans showed differences in leg length and bone density, the patient's ability to bear weight on the treated leg improved significantly. This case shows that combining these advanced techniques can be a good approach for treating complex fractures in veterinary practice.

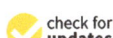

Citation: Bae, M.; Kang, B.-J.; Kim, J. Application of Hybrid External Skeletal Fixation with Bone Tissue Engineering Techniques for Comminuted Fracture of the Proximal Radius in a Dog. *Animals* **2024**, *14*, 3480. https://doi.org/10.3390/ani14233480

Academic Editors: L. Miguel Carreira, João Alves, Rachel C. Murray and Christophe R. Casteleyn

Received: 22 August 2024
Revised: 12 November 2024
Accepted: 28 November 2024
Published: 2 December 2024

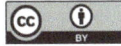

Copyright: © 2024 by the authors. Licensee MDPI, Basel, Switzerland. This article is an open access article distributed under the terms and conditions of the Creative Commons Attribution (CC BY) license (https://creativecommons.org/licenses/by/4.0/).

Abstract: A seven-month-old male Pomeranian presented with left forelimb lameness after a fall. Radiographic assessment confirmed proximal radial head and ulnar comminuted fracture. The initial surgical intervention involved the use of hybrid external skeletal fixation (ESF) to stabilize the radial head, concomitant with the application of a composite of bone morphogenetic protein type 2 (BMP-2)-loaded hydroxyapatite and gelatin microparticles at the fracture site. Although successful radial head healing was achieved, the ESF pinholes caused a defect in the proximal ulnar diaphysis. Subsequently, the ESF was removed, and a locking plate was applied in conjunction with the BMP-2-loaded collagen membrane to correct the radius defect. Clinical follow-up at 4.8 years postoperatively revealed a mildly decreased range of motion of the affected elbow joint, but no clinical symptoms such as lameness. Radiography revealed minimal degenerative changes and a radioulnar synostosis. Computed tomography revealed differences in the leg length and bone density. Gait analysis revealed that the left forelimb had a significant improvement in weight-bearing capacity based on weight distribution–peak vertical force metrics, compared with the right forelimb. Based on clinical outcomes, the combined application of hybrid ESF and bone tissue engineering techniques can be considered a feasible alternative treatment for radial head fractures.

Keywords: radial head fracture; bone tissue engineering; hybrid ESF; gait analysis; canine

1. Introduction

The prevailing fracture sites of small and toy breed dogs regarding age and body size are as follows: radius/ulna, tibia, femur, and humerus [1–3]. The radius and ulna are relatively thin and long in small and toy breed dogs, making fractures more common when excessive pressure is applied to their forelimbs, particularly during activities such as jumping, or following external impacts such as falls. Most radial and ulnar fractures occur in the distal region, whereas fractures in the proximal region are less common. Proximal radial fractures are rare and challenging to access surgically because of anatomical constraints [4]. Although internal fixation provides greater stability in typical proximal radial transverse fractures, placement of implants onto the radial head becomes challenging in cases of more comminuted radial head and neck fractures. In such situations, external skeletal fixation (ESF) devices can be employed as a surgical approach [3,5,6].

ESF offers the advantage of minimizing soft tissue damage, making it an effective option for fractures in regions with relatively little soft tissue [7–10]. Additionally, the surgeon can apply a bilateral or biplane frame to further stabilize the fracture. The hybrid ESF technique, which combines both linear and circular external fixation components, is commonly recommended for fractures involving the juxta-articular bone segments near the joints. This is particularly valuable in cases where the application of plate screws is challenging [7]. Furthermore, in cases of complex fractures affecting the radial head and neck, the use of a hybrid ESF may be indicated to float the radial head and maintain its position, utilizing a linear ESF that secures the olecranon proximally and the radius distally, thereby allowing the radial head to be floated and stabilized by the surrounding soft tissues [4].

In recent years, extensive research has been conducted in the fields of tissue engineering and regenerative medicine to identify methods for enhancing bone healing [11,12]. Bone tissue engineering (BTE) focuses on the development of innovative biomedical techniques to treat skeletal injuries and is a promising treatment method for animals with fractures. BTE strategies involve the application of bone grafts to a scaffold, which are subsequently implanted in vivo to target bone defects; however, its long-term outcomes have not been sufficiently characterized yet.

To the authors' knowledge, there are currently no documented cases in the veterinary field that apply hybrid ESF in conjunction with BTE for fractures of the proximal radius, and no cases have confirmed the bone status through long-term follow-up after the application of BTE. This paper reports the bone status and gait of a small breed dog treated with hybrid ESF using BTE techniques 4.8 years after the procedure.

2. Case Description

A 7-month-old, 3.3 kg, intact male Pomeranian suffered a complex fracture of the left proximal radius and ulna after falling. A tie-in IM pin was placed to fix the fracture at a private veterinary clinic; however, the fixation failed, and the fracture recurred. At referral, the patient could not weight-bear on the left forelimb during the standing physical examination. For subjective evaluation, the clinical lameness scores were used, which were based on six factors such as lameness score, range of motion (ROM), and pain, with each factor evaluated on a scale of 1 to 4 or 5 points (total score range: 6 to 27) [13]. Assessment using the clinical lameness score criteria revealed 24 points out of 27 points. Radiographs revealed poor bone healing due to the previous pin fixation and a comminuted fracture of the left proximal radius and ulna (Figure 1A). As the fracture was near the radial head, the bone structure was not clearly visible on radiography, necessitating a computed tomography (CT) scan for accurate fracture assessment and appropriate surgical planning. CT revealed a proximal non-reducible radial head fracture, which was fractured into three proximal fragments (6.5 mm × 5.9 mm, 7.5 mm × 2.9 mm, 10.4 mm × 4.1 mm), along with a proximal ulnar fracture (Figure 1B). Articular surface damage was also observed. Based on comprehensive examination, it was determined that stabilizing the radial head was essential to preserve the affected forelimb. Due to the radial head's non-reducible fracture, direct stabilization through implant fixation was not feasible. Therefore, as a surgical treatment strategy, it was decided to apply a type II hybrid ESF, combining a bilateral uniplanar linear system with an Ilizarov-type circular system, to create space for the placement of two screws on the radial head.

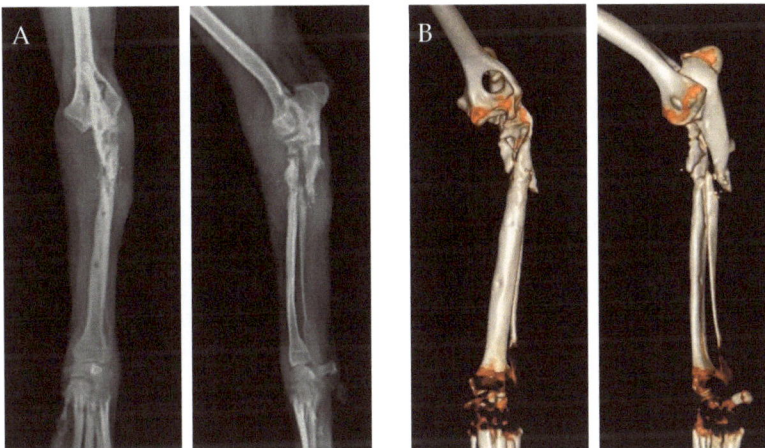

Figure 1. (**A**) Preoperative radiography image. (**B**) Preoperative computed tomography reconstruction image.

2.1. Surgical Treatment I

After obtaining a CT image of the left forelimb, a 3D anatomical model was fabricated for preoperative planning and surgical rehearsal using an ESF device.

The first surgical treatment was performed one week after referral (Figure 2A–C). The patient was premedicated with 0.2 mg/kg of intravenous (IV) midazolam (midazolam, Inj®; Bukwang Pharm, Seoul, Republic of Korea). Anesthesia was induced with 6 mg/kg of IV propofol (Anepol, Inj®; Hana Pharm, Seoul, Republic of Korea) and maintained with inhaled isoflurane (Ifran; Hana Pharm, Seoul, Republic of Korea) in oxygen. Cefazolin (Cefazolin, Inj®; Chong Kun Dang Pharm, Seoul, Republic of Korea) a prophylactic antimicrobial agent, was administered before surgery and intraoperatively at an initial dose of 25 mg/kg IV, with repeat doses every 90 min throughout the procedure. The dog was positioned in lateral recumbency, with the affected limb placed in the uppermost position. The skin was aseptically prepared for surgery. After palpating the olecranon, a craniomedial skin incision was made at the proximal radius. Proximal radial defects were observed, and a predesigned hybrid ESF (IMEX™ Veterinary, Inc., Longview, TX, USA) was applied, combining type II linear ESF at the proximal site of the fracture and two circular ESFs at the distal site of the fracture. The linear ESF was equipped with six connecting clamps and fixation pins in the form of sequential wires (1.0 mm, 0.9 mm, and 1.0 mm) from the most proximal to the distal part of the olecranon. Circular ESFs were implanted using two 0.9 mm k-wires at a distal radius. A bone graft mixture comprising recombinant human bone morphogenetic protein type-2 (rhBMP-2) (0.25 mg; NOVOSIS, Seoul, Republic of Korea) loaded with hydroxyapatite (HA) and gelatin microparticles (GMP) was inserted into the defect site to expedite bone healing. The dosage of rhBMP-2 was determined as described by Massie et al. [14]. After insertion of the bone graft, the muscles and skin layers were closed routinely. Postoperatively, cephalexin (Phalexin capsules, Donghwa Pharm, Seoul, Republic of Korea) was administered at 25 mg/kg q12h PO for 5 days. Postoperative analgesia involved intermittent tramadol 4 mg/kg PO (Tridol, Yuhan Pharm, Seoul, Republic of Korea) as necessary. Meloxicam (Metacam, Boehringer Ingelheim, Seoul, Republic of Korea) was administered at 0.2 mg/kg IV on the day of surgery followed by 0.1 mg/kg PO starting 24 h after surgery for 14 days.

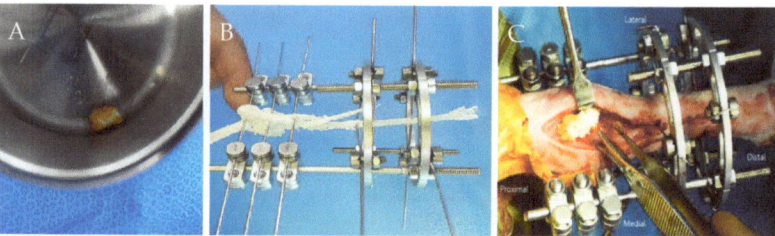

Figure 2. Intraoperative images taken during the first surgery. (**A**) Gelatin microparticle (GMP) loaded with BMP-2; (**B**) simulation of the external skeletal fixation (ESF) device on a 3D-printed model; (**C**) insertion of the BMP-2 loaded HA and GMP mixture at the radius defect site.

2.2. Surgical Treatment II

One month after the first surgery, radiography revealed bone regeneration at the radial head. Two months following surgery, bone continuity and sufficient size (18.8 mm × 7.5 mm) of the proximal radial head fragment for screw placement were observed. However, loosening of the proximal pins and widening of the ESF pinholes were also noted, leading to the decision that revision surgery was necessary.

The anesthesia protocol was identical to that used in the previous surgery. A craniomedial incision was made to access the surgical site, elevate the extensor carpi radialis muscle, and separate it from the supinator muscle using a periosteal elevator. In the initial procedure of the second surgery, a segment of the previously implanted bone-substitute material and adjacent bone tissue from the proximal radial head were harvested while trimming the callus that had formed on the radial surface as part of the bone healing process, prior to plate application for internal fixation. A collagen membrane loaded with rhBMP-2 was placed around the defective area to enhance osteogenesis. Fracture fixation was subsequently performed using a locking plate (24-holes 2.0 mm, straight plate, ARIX Vet) (Figure 3A–C). The supinator muscle was then sutured to the surrounding muscles, and the skin layers were closed routinely.

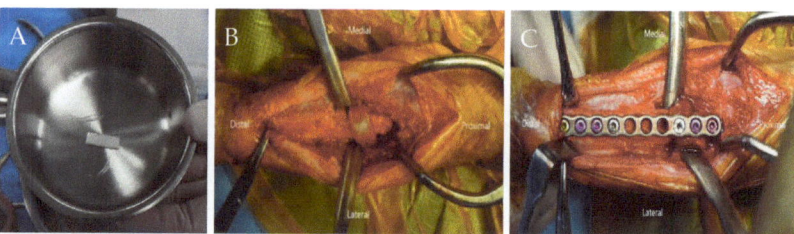

Figure 3. Intraoperative images of the second surgery. (**A**) The collagen membrane loaded with BMP-2; (**B**) a collagen membrane covering the radius defect area; (**C**) locking plate fixation of the radius.

2.3. Statistical Data Analysis

All data were analyzed with GraphPad Prism 10 (GraphPad Software, Inc., La Jolla, CA, USA). The HU values of the affected and contralateral radii were compared using the Mann–Whitney U test. The gait analysis data were analyzed with a repeated measures analysis of variance (ANOVA) followed by a post hoc Šídák multiple comparisons test. Statistical significance was defined as $p < 0.05$.

2.4. Diagnostic Assessment and Outcomes

One month after the first surgery, radiographic evaluation revealed bone regeneration of the radial head, with maintenance of the ESF and connection of the proximal three fragments. Two months after surgery, the upper radial head formed a single segment (18.8 mm × 7.5 mm), allowing sufficient space for plate fixation, even without hybrid

ESF. Therefore, a revision surgery was performed using plate fixation to correct the radius defects and provide a more stable biomechanical environment for the healing bone.

The bone specimens harvested during the revision surgery were histologically processed with hematoxylin and eosin (H&E) and Masson's trichrome (MT) staining to evaluate the regenerated bone tissue morphology. In histological analysis of bone regeneration, H&E staining revealed newly formed bone tissue around the HA, with osteoblasts and osteoclasts observed at the HA border (Figure 4A). MT staining of the same area revealed that immature bone tissue was stained blue, whereas mature bone tissue rarely stained brick red (Figure 4B).

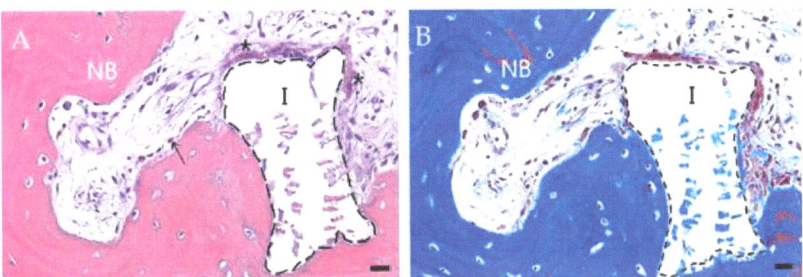

Figure 4. Results of histological analysis at three months after BMP-2 loaded HA and GMP mixture insertion. (**A**) H&E staining, (**B**) Masson's trichrome staining image showing a section of the bone fragment. I: implant (black dotted lines). NB: new bone. Arrow: osteoblast. Asterisks: osteoclast. Scale bar: 20 μm.

Two weeks after the second surgery, the ROM of the affected limb's elbow joint was found to be mildly reduced by 10–20% compared to that of the normal limb. Radiography revealed that the radial head was positioned below the typical location, resulting in decreased joint congruity. However, the overall condition of the joint improved compared to that at the initial visit, and continuity of the bone within the defect areas was observed. Five weeks after the second surgery, partial recovery of the asymmetrical gait was revealed. Nine weeks after the second surgery, the patient's gait had improved, and the clinical lameness score criteria revealed 8 points out of 27 points.

At the 4.8 years long-term follow-up visit, the owner reported no forelimb-related clinical signs such as lameness. Radiographically, evidence of synostosis between the proximal ulna and radius along with mild osteoarthritis were observed in the affected elbow joint (Figure 5). Furthermore, on CT, while the lengths of both humeri were nearly the same, the right radius was 83.5 mm and the left radius was 70 mm, meaning that the length of the affected limb was approximately 17% shorter than that of the normal limb.

CT was performed to compare and evaluate the bone properties of the contralateral and affected radii (window level, 450 HU; window width, 4500 HU). Based on the 3D reconstructed images of the patient's normal radius and the surgically treated radius, the Hounsfield unit (HU) value was measured at 70–80% of the distal to proximal length of the affected forelimb where the bone graft was implanted. The cross-sectional areas of the bones were concurrently measured. For the normal radius, the HU measurements were obtained at the same level as those for the affected radius (Figure 6A). In addition, a region-of-interest tool was used to measure the HU at the midpoints of the cortices (C_{med}, C_{lat}, C_{cran}, and C_{caud}). The HU values of the normal bone tissue on the right side were significantly higher than those in the area with bone graft insertion ($p < 0.0001$) (Figure 6B).

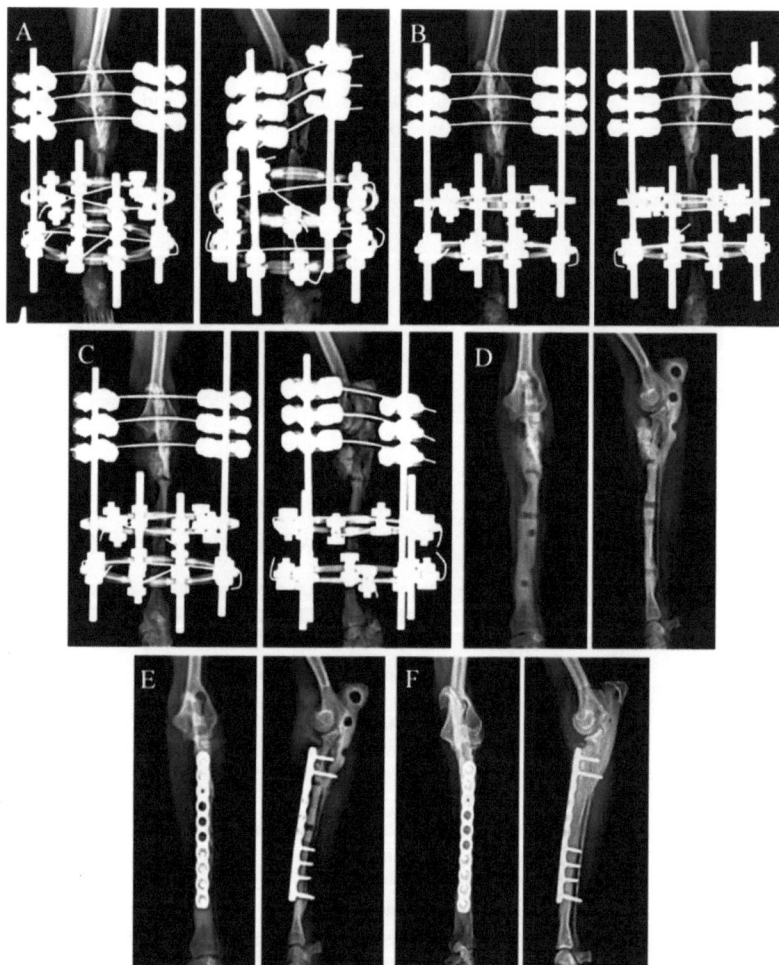

Figure 5. Sequential radiographic images are shown at 0 days (**A**), 4 weeks (**B**), and 8 weeks (**C**) after fixation of the hybrid ESF with bone graft materials. (**D**) Due to ESF pin hole defects, plate fixation with bone graft materials was performed at 12 weeks (**E**). Radiography showing radioulnar synostosis (**F**) 4.8 years after the insertion of the plate.

The gait analysis after the second surgery was objectively evaluated using a pressure sensor walkway (Walkway, Tekscan Inc., Norwood, MA, USA), and the symmetry index (SI) and weight distribution (WD) were assessed using the data obtained from Tekscan software (Walkway 7.66). The gait analysis results at 12 days, 5 weeks, and 4.8 years post second surgery revealed a reduction in the difference between the peak vertical force (PVF) and vertical impulse (VI) for both forelimbs (Figure 7). Compared with pre-operative values, the SI and WD analysis showed an increase in both PVF and VI in the affected limb (one-way RM ANOVA, $p < 0.0001$). Additionally, the SI-PVF value became negative, indicating an increase in the PVF of the left limb compared with that of the right limb. This suggests an improvement in walking ability at 4.8 years post second surgery.

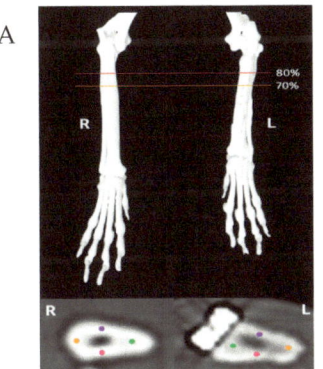 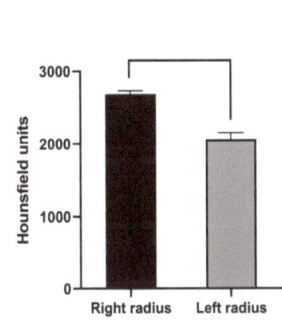

Figure 6. (**A**) Measurement of the Hounsfield unit (HU) values in 70–80% of the distal to proximal length of the affected radius and the same level of the right radius from CT images. Bone mineral density was estimated from HU measurement at the cranial (purple), caudal (pink), medial (green), and lateral (orange) cortices. The mean cross-sectional BMD was calculated. (**B**) A significant difference in the mean HU value between bilateral radii can be observed.

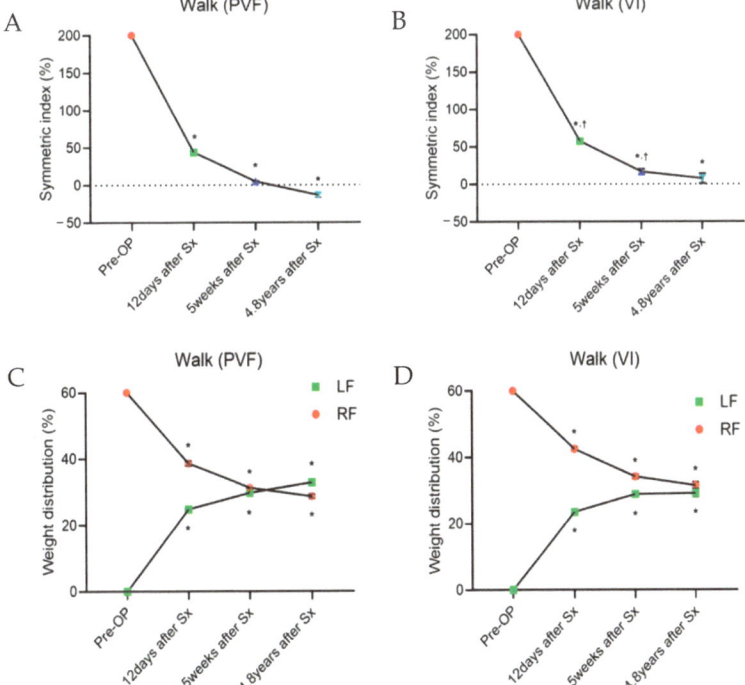

Figure 7. Gait analysis of the pressure sensor walkway. (**A,B**) The symmetry index of the left forelimb decreased after fixation of the radius locking plate (2nd Surgery). (**C,D**) Weight distribution of the bilateral limbs revealed a tendency towards restoration of the left forelimb function. PVF: peak vertical force; VI: vertical impulse; RF: right forelimb; LF: left forelimb; * significant change from pre-operation; † significant change from 12 days after fixation of radius locking plate.

3. Discussion

Stabilization of complex fractures involving small segments near the joint can be challenging. The length and shape of the fractured segment must be carefully considered during the fixation. Otherwise, instances such as very short proximal segments may not provide sufficient space for internal fixation [4,7]. Alternatively, procedures such as radial head ostectomy or elbow arthrodesis are available as salvage interventions [15–18]. ESF is an effective treatment for the minimally invasive correction and fixation of complex tibia and radius fractures [8]. The Ilizarov method of circular ESF is commonly used for angular limb deformity correction, limb lengthening, and complex juxta-articular fractures. Nevertheless, considering the angle of the elbow joint in a normal standing position, a pure Ilizarov full ring frame may impede elbow movement, which could negatively affect joint mobility during recovery. To minimize interference with elbow flexion, specific rings such as "stretch" or "partial" rings could be used at the proximal part of the frame. However, in the case of juxta-articular fractures of the upper portion of the radius, applying hybrid ESF, which combines the advantages of both linear and circular ESF, may provide a more beneficial solution. Linear ESF offers static axial stiffness for fractures near the joint in the proximal region where screw insertion for plate fixation is challenging. The application of fine-wire fixation to a circular ring further provides strong stability to small bone fragments. Moreover, tensioned wires crossing the ring offer rigid fixation while generating nonlinear dynamic axial micromotion at the fracture site, promoting faster callus formation compared to conventional healing. Furthermore, fixation wires offer multiple fixation points even for extremely small bone fragments [7,10,19]. However, while hybrid ESF provides significant advantages, their overall weight may restrict functional ambulation in underweight patients. Although manufacturers produce systems specifically designed for miniature and small breeds, it is advisable to consider replacing conventional fixators with lighter alternatives, such as acrylic ESF, to maintain comparable biomechanical efficacy while alleviating the mechanical load on low-body-weight patients [4,20]. A hybrid linear-circular ESF can be used to bridge the antebrachium using a hybrid rod attached to the ring, which enables the placement of transfixation pins on the lateral side of the olecranon and extends to the radius and ulna, distal to the fracture site. This method allows the proximal radius to 'float', while still being attached to the ulna by ligaments and a joint capsule to maintain its position [4,21]. As the proximal radial region is relatively stable owing to the ulna and ligaments, inserting linear pins into the olecranon and affixing the ring to the distal radius could provide stability. In this case, a hybrid ESF was utilized to preserve the radius without directly stabilizing the fracture site, allowing for temporary floating of the radial head. Although this method aids in maintaining the position of the fractured radial head, the successful union of the fragmented radial head remains uncertain. Consequently, tissue engineering techniques may be considered to enhance bone regeneration and facilitate successful healing.

Bone tissue can regenerate naturally following minor damage without exceeding the critical size threshold. However, substantial defects beyond this threshold require clinical intervention for functional recovery and eventual complete healing [22,23]. The application of bone fixation plates, bone allografts, or autografts is the standard treatment for substantial bone defects [24]. Despite these approaches, concerns regarding the necessity for subsequent removal and the potential side effects persist. The BTE strategy aims to develop materials that promote bone regeneration at defect sites without causing these problems [25]. These biomaterials promote bone regeneration through one or more of the following processes: osteoinduction, osteoconduction, or osteogenesis. In orthopedic defects of load-bearing anatomical sites, such as long bones, the development of new bone tissue must occur quickly to alleviate pain. It is preferable to use osteoconductive materials that provide a three-dimensional structure at the defect site along with osteoinductive materials that induce ossification [26]. In this case, HA and BMP-2 were applied as osteoconductive and osteoinductive materials, respectively (Figure 2). HA ($Ca_{10}(PO_4)_6(OH)_2$) fills the void space at the implant site while providing a three-dimensional structure that allows the growth of the microvasculature, surrounding tissues, and osteoprogenitors into the bone interior [27,28]. BMP-2 stimulates the differentiation and proliferation of mesenchymal stem cells into osteoblasts, thereby promoting bone formation, maturation, and ossification [25]. However, the direct administration of high doses of BMP-2 can lead to side effects, including osteoclast activation and inflammatory responses [14]. Furthermore, as bone healing occurs over several months, it is crucial that BMP-2 be released slowly. Experimental studies [29,30] have demonstrated successful bone regeneration through the utilization of BMP-2-loaded GMP and a collagen membrane, inducing sustained release of BMP-2, thus facilitating osteogenesis. Woven bone with irregular collagen fibers is immature and typically found in developing bones and fracture healing sites. This material is subsequently replaced by lamellar bone, comprising of organized collagen layers [31]. In this case, histological analysis with H&E and MT staining revealed regions of bone matrix containing both irregularly woven and multilayered lamellar bone (Figure 4). The presence of blood vessels and bone cells such as osteoblasts and osteoclasts suggests active bone remodeling, growth, and maintenance in areas where HA is present [28,32]. The observed histological evidence supports the osteoconductive properties of HA and osteoinductive properties of BMP-2 at the fracture site, promoting osteogenesis and bone regeneration.

CT is increasingly recognized as a valuable tool for the noninvasive measurement of bone mineral density, utilizing the HU scale based on the standard linear attenuation coefficient [33,34]. For the quantitative assessment based on CT images, the HU values were measured at the midpoints of the cortices (Figure 6A). In this present case, radioulnar synostosis (Figure 5F), a common complication of radioulnar fracture repair in dogs and cats was observed, resulting in an inconsistent bone shape. CT examination revealed that the affected radius had lower HU values than the opposite forelimb. In addition, the cross-sectional area of the distal left radius, where there was no plate, was larger than the corresponding area of the right radius. Lower HU values and increased cross-sectional areas were observed because the left forelimb was 17% shorter than the right forelimb, as shown in the CT scan. Generally, leg length discrepancy results in shorter leg dragging during walking, leading to increased vertical movement of the center of gravity and, consequently, increased energy consumption [35]. Stress refers to the resistance within bone tissue that develops in response to loads such as compression, bending, and torsion applied to the bone. According to Wolff's law, when a specific bone is subjected to increased loads, it remodels over time to become stronger and to withstand such loads, resulting in increased bone thickness [34,36]. Bone density depends on the applied load; a decreased load leads to decreased density and can cause osteoporosis over time. When a plate with a high Young's modulus is used to fix a fractured bone, the load is transferred to the plate, thereby altering the stress distribution. This reduces bone stress, causing stress shielding, which decreases bone density and elasticity, progressively weakening the bone [37,38]. In this case, surgery was performed at the age of 1, a highly active age, allowing the bone to experience a significant load-bearing environment as walking improved postoperatively. To adapt to the increased vertical movement of the center of gravity and the resulting increase in impact, the left radius was speculated to have thickened and strengthened. However, the lower HU values on the left side of the CT scan were attributed to the plate causing less stress to the bone, leading to the activation of osteoclasts that perceived unnecessary bone tissue, resulting in a relative decrease in bone density.

Recently, gait analysis has been increasingly applied to objectively detect and monitor lameness in small animals with musculoskeletal or neurological disorders [39,40]. In this case, kinetic gait analysis based on paw pressure was used to assess postoperative gait. At 12 and 5 weeks after the second surgery (Figure 7), the differences in the PVF and VI between the affected and normal limbs tended to decrease, approaching an SI of zero. At 4.8 years, distinctive gait characteristics of the shorter left limb were observed, including increased vertical displacement of the center of mass and decreased stance time, stride length, and walking speed [35]. The patient also exhibited these characteristics in the shorter left forelimb, resulting in an increased PVF and decreased VI. Consequently, the

SI-PVF value becomes negative, whereas the SI-VI value remains positive. At 4.8 years, the absolute mean values of SI-PVF and SI-VI were 3.53% and 11.64%, respectively. Even in healthy dogs, there can be a maximum of <6% asymmetry between limbs [41]. The SI generally records the differences between normal and pathological gaits and evaluates changes in asymmetry due to enhanced pathological conditions [42]. Although the SI-VI value was relatively more asymmetric, owing to the reduced stance time of the left limb compared to that of the normal limb, the SI-PVF fell within the range of asymmetry observed in normal dogs.

This study has several limitations. First, as we presented only a single case, additional prospective studies are required to validate the feasibility and repeatability of the hybrid ESF and BTE techniques in promoting proper bone regeneration. The use of threaded pins, which offer better bone holding power, is recommended for linear ESF applications [43]. Unfortunately, smooth pins were used in this study, and periodic monitoring was conducted to minimize potential instability. Despite the non-ideal pins, BMP-2 was applied to the fracture site, resulting in successful bone healing. Furthermore, fusion of the radius and ulna occurred after the procedure, resulting in impaired physiological joint movements. This complication has also been reported in previous studies [21], highlighting the need for further investigations to prevent such complications. In addition, it is possible to consider removing the screws while checking the bone density through periodic monitoring.

4. Conclusions

In conclusion, the patient experienced a radial head fracture during the growth period. Long-term follow-up revealed complications, including decreased joint congruity, radioulnar synostosis, and arthritis development. Despite these issues, joint preservation remains a meaningful outcome. However, it is important to recognize that this is based on a single clinical case and may not be widely applicable without further research. Additionally, the patient's low body weight likely contributed to an easier adaptation to biomechanics. The successful application of hybrid ESF and BTE techniques to unite complex radial head fractures and defects highlights the potential of this approach as a viable treatment option, prioritizing joint preservation over salvage interventions.

Author Contributions: M.B.: writing—original draft preparation, writing—review and editing; B.-J.K.: conceptualization, writing—review and editing; J.K.: supervision, methodology, writing—review and editing. All authors have read and agreed to the published version of the manuscript.

Funding: This research was funded by the Basic Science Research Program through the National Research Foundation of Korea (NRF) funded by the Ministry of Education (RS-2023-00210585) and by 2023 Research Grant from Kangwon National University.

Institutional Review Board Statement: Ethical review and approval were not required as we report a case study from a veterinary medical teaching hospital. We have the consent of both the owner and veterinarian that this dog (which underwent the listed examinations and surgical intervention) was treated not for an experimental but for a medical reason.

Informed Consent Statement: Informed consent was obtained from all subjects involved in the study. The patient was a client-owned animal and written informed consent was obtained from the owner of the animal.

Data Availability Statement: All relevant data is contained within the article, the original contributions presented in the study are included in the article. Further inquiries can be directed to the corresponding author.

Conflicts of Interest: The authors declare that the study was conducted in the absence of any commercial or financial relationships that could be construed as potential conflicts of interest.

References

1. Roush, J.K. *Prevalence of Bone Fractures in Dogs and Cats, July/August 2015 ed.*; Today's Veterinary Practice: Gainesville, FL, USA, 2015; Volume 2015.
2. Piras, L.; Cappellari, F.; Peirone, B.; Ferretti, A. Treatment of Fractures of the Distal Radius and Ulna in Toy Breed Dogs with Circular External Skeletal Fixation: A Retrospective Study. *Vet. Comp. Orthop. Traumatol.* **2011**, *24*, 228–235. [CrossRef] [PubMed]
3. Kang, B.-J.; Ryu, H.-H.; Park, S.; Kim, Y.; Kweon, O.-K.; Hayashi, K. Clinical Evaluation of a Mini Locking Plate System for Fracture Repair of the Radius and Ulna in Miniature Breed Dogs. *Vet. Comp. Orthop. Traumatol.* **2016**, *29*, 522–527. [CrossRef] [PubMed]
4. Johnston, S.A.; Tobias, K.M. *Veterinary Surgery: Small Animal Expert Consult-E-Book: 2-Volume Set*; Elsevier Health Sciences: Amsterdam, The Netherlands, 2017.
5. Gatineau, M.; Planté, J. Ulnar Interlocking Intramedullary Nail Stabilization of a Proximal Radio-Ulnar Fracture in a Dog. *Vet. Surg.* **2010**, *39*, 1025–1029. [CrossRef] [PubMed]
6. Johnson, A.L.; Kneller, S.; Weigel, R. Radial and Tibial Fracture Repair with External Skeletal Fixation: Effects of Fracture Type, Reduction, and Complications on Healing. *Vet. Surg.* **1989**, *18*, 367–372. [CrossRef] [PubMed]
7. Farese, J.P.; Lewis, D.D.; Cross, A.R.; Collins, K.E.; Anderson, G.M.; Halling, K.B. Use of IMEX SK-Circular External Fixator Hybrid Constructs for Fracture Stabilization in Dogs and Cats. *J. Am. Anim. Hosp. Assoc.* **2002**, *38*, 279–289. [CrossRef]
8. Laverty, P.; Johnson, A.; Toombs, J.; Schaeffer, D. Simple and Multiple Fractures of the Radius Treated with an External Fixator. *Vet. Comp. Orthop. Traumatol.* **2002**, *15*, 97–103. [CrossRef]
9. Marcellin-Little, D.J. Fracture Treatment with Circular External Fixation. *Vet. Clin. Small Anim. Pract.* **1999**, *29*, 1153–1170. [CrossRef]
10. Johnson, A.; Schaeffer, D. Evolution of the Treatment of Canine Radial and Tibial Fractures with External Fixators. *Vet. Comp. Orthop. Traumatol.* **2008**, *21*, 256–261. [CrossRef]
11. Kempen, D.H.; Lu, L.; Hefferan, T.E.; Creemers, L.B.; Maran, A.; Classic, K.L.; Dhert, W.J.; Yaszemski, M.J. Retention of In Vitro and In Vivo BMP-2 Bioactivities in Sustained Delivery Vehicles for Bone Tissue Engineering. *Biomaterials* **2008**, *29*, 3245–3252. [CrossRef]
12. Rosen, V. BMP2 Signaling in Bone Development and Repair. *Cytokine Growth Factor. Rev.* **2009**, *20*, 475–480. [CrossRef]
13. Lee, M.-I.; Kim, J.-H.; Kwak, H.-H.; Woo, H.-M.; Han, J.-H.; Yayon, A.; Jung, Y.-C.; Cho, J.-M.; Kang, B.-J. A Placebo-Controlled Study Comparing the Efficacy of Intra-Articular Injections of Hyaluronic Acid and a Novel Hyaluronic Acid-Platelet-Rich Plasma Conjugate in a Canine Model of Osteoarthritis. *J. Orthop. Surg. Res.* **2019**, *14*, 1–12. [CrossRef]
14. Massie, A.M.; Kapatkin, A.S.; Fuller, M.C.; Verstraete, F.J.; Arzi, B. Outcome of Nonunion Fractures in Dogs Treated with Fixation, Compression Resistant Matrix, and Recombinant Human Bone Morphogenetic Protein-2. *Vet. Comp. Orthop. Traumatol.* **2017**, *30*, 153–159. [CrossRef] [PubMed]
15. McCarthy, J.; Comerford, E.J.; Innes, J.F.; Pettitt, R.A. Elbow Arthrodesis Using a Medially Positioned Plate in 6 Dogs. *Vet. Comp. Orthop. Traumatol.* **2020**, *33*, 051–058. [CrossRef] [PubMed]
16. Heidenreich, D.; Fourie, Y.; Barreau, P. Presumptive Congenital Radial Head Sub-Luxation in a Shih Tzu: Successful Management by Radial Head Ostectomy. *J. Small Anim. Pract.* **2015**, *56*, 626–629. [CrossRef]
17. Kim, J.; Song, J.; Kim, S.-Y.; Kang, B.-J. Single Oblique Osteotomy for Correction of Congenital Radial Head Luxation with Concurrent Complex Angular Limb Deformity in a Dog: A Case Report. *J. Vet. Sci.* **2020**, *21*, e62. [CrossRef] [PubMed]
18. Sjöström, L.; Kasström, H.; Källberg, M. Ununited Anconeal Process in the Dog. Pathogenesis and Treatment by Osteotomy of the Ulna. *Vet. Comp. Orthop. Traumatol.* **1995**, *8*, 170–176. [CrossRef]
19. Clarke, S.; Carmichael, S. Treatment of Distal Diaphyseal Fractures Using Hybrid External Skeletal Fixation in Three Dogs. *J. Small Anim. Pract.* **2006**, *47*, 98–103. [CrossRef]
20. Tyagi, S.K.; Aithal, H.P.; Kinjavdekar, P.; Amarpal, S.; Pawde, A.M.; Srivastava, T.; Singh, J.; Madhu, D.N. In Vitro Biomechanical Testing of Different Configurations of Acrylic External Skeletal Fixator Constructs. *Vet. Comp. Orthop. Traumatol.* **2015**, *28*, 227–233. [CrossRef]
21. Vezzoni, L.; Abrescia, P.; Vezzoni, A. Internal Radioulnar Fixation for Treatment of Nonunion of Proximal Radius and Ulna Fractures in a Toy Breed Dog. *VCOT Open* **2021**, *4*, e24–e31. [CrossRef]
22. Schemitsch, E.H. Size Matters: Defining Critical in Bone Defect Size! *J. Orthop. Trauma* **2017**, *31*, S20–S22. [CrossRef]
23. Annamalai, R.T.; Hong, X.; Schott, N.G.; Tiruchinapally, G.; Levi, B.; Stegemann, J.P. Injectable Osteogenic Microtissues Containing Mesenchymal Stromal Cells Conformally Fill and Repair Critical-Size Defects. *Biomaterials* **2019**, *208*, 32–44. [CrossRef] [PubMed]
24. Alghazali, K.M.; Nima, Z.A.; Hamzah, R.N.; Dhar, M.S.; Anderson, D.E.; Biris, A.S. Bone-Tissue Engineering: Complex Tunable Structural and Biological Responses to Injury, Drug Delivery, and Cell-Based Therapies. *Drug Metab. Rev.* **2015**, *47*, 431–454. [CrossRef] [PubMed]
25. Winkler, T.; Sass, F.; Duda, G.; Schmidt-Bleek, K. A Review of Biomaterials in Bone Defect Healing, Remaining Shortcomings and Future Opportunities for Bone Tissue Engineering: The Unsolved Challenge. *Bone Jt. Res.* **2018**, *7*, 232–243. [CrossRef] [PubMed]
26. Boden, S.D. Overview of the Biology of Lumbar Spine Fusion and Principles for Selecting a Bone Graft Substitute. *Spine* **2002**, *27*, S26–S31. [CrossRef] [PubMed]
27. Son, J.; Kim, J.; Lee, K.; Hwang, J.; Choi, Y.; Seo, Y.; Jeon, H.; Kang, H.C.; Woo, H.-M.; Kang, B.-J. DNA Aptamer Immobilized Hydroxyapatite for Enhancing Angiogenesis and Bone Regeneration. *Acta Biomater.* **2019**, *99*, 469–478. [CrossRef]

28. Attia, M.S.; Mohammed, H.M.; Attia, M.G.; Hamid, M.A.A.E.; Shoeriabah, E.A. Histological and Histomorphometric Evaluation of Hydroxyapatite-Based Biomaterials in Surgically Created Defects Around Implants in Dogs. *J. Periodontol.* **2019**, *90*, 281–287. [CrossRef] [PubMed]
29. Kim, S.; Kim, J.; Gajendiran, M.; Yoon, M.; Hwang, M.P.; Wang, Y.; Kang, B.-J.; Kim, K. Enhanced Skull Bone Regeneration by Sustained Release of BMP-2 in Interpenetrating Composite Hydrogels. *Biomacromolecules* **2018**, *19*, 4239–4249. [CrossRef] [PubMed]
30. Yamamoto, M.; Takahashi, Y.; Tabata, Y. Controlled Release by Biodegradable Hydrogels Enhances the Ectopic Bone Formation of Bone Morphogenetic Protein. *Biomaterials* **2003**, *24*, 4375–4383. [CrossRef] [PubMed]
31. Shapiro, F. Bone Development and Its Relation to Fracture Repair. The Role of Mesenchymal Osteoblasts and Surface Osteoblasts. *Eur. Cell Mater.* **2008**, *15*, e76. [CrossRef] [PubMed]
32. Lee, J.-S.; Park, W.-Y.; Cha, J.-K.; Jung, U.-W.; Kim, C.-S.; Lee, Y.-K.; Choi, S.-H. Periodontal Tissue Reaction to Customized Nano-Hydroxyapatite Block Scaffold in One-Wall Intrabony Defect: A Histologic Study in Dogs. *J. Periodontal Implant. Sci.* **2012**, *42*, 50–58. [CrossRef]
33. Mejia, S.; Iodence, A.; Griffin, L.; Withrow, S.; Puttlitz, C.; Salman, M.; Seguin, B. Comparison of Cross-Sectional Geometrical Properties and Bone Density of the Proximal Radius Between Saint Bernard and Other Giant Breed Dogs. *Vet. Surg.* **2019**, *48*, 947–955. [CrossRef] [PubMed]
34. Hamish, R.; Denny, S.J.B. *A Guide to Canine and Feline Orthopaedic Surgery*; Willey: Hoboken, NJ, USA, 2008.
35. Gurney, B. Leg length discrepancy. *Gait Posture* **2002**, *15*, 195–206. [CrossRef] [PubMed]
36. Boyle, C.; Kim, I.Y. Three-Dimensional Micro-Level Computational Study of Wolff's Law Via Trabecular Bone Remodeling in the Human Proximal Femur Using Design Space Topology Optimization. *J. Biomech.* **2011**, *44*, 935–942. [CrossRef]
37. Fouda, N.; Mostafa, R.; Saker, A. Numerical Study of Stress Shielding Reduction at Fractured Bone Using Metallic and Composite Bone-Plate Models. *Ain. Shams Eng. J.* **2019**, *10*, 481–488. [CrossRef]
38. Raffa, M.L.; Nguyen, V.H.; Hernigou, P.; Flouzat-Lachaniette, C.H.; Haiat, G. Stress Shielding at the Bone-Implant Interface: Influence of Surface Roughness and of the Bone-Implant Contact Ratio. *J. Orthop. Res.* **2021**, *39*, 1174–1183. [CrossRef]
39. Miles, J.; Nielsen, M.; Mouritzen, A.; Pedersen, T.; Nielsen, L.N.; Vitger, A.; Poulsen, H.H. Gait Analysis of Lameness-Free Dogs: Experience with a Tekscan Pressure-Sensitive Walkway System. In *BSAVA Congress Proceedings 2019*; BSAVA Library: Gloucester, UK, 2019; p. 521.
40. Duerr, F. *Canine Lameness*; John Wiley & Sons: Hoboken, NJ, USA, 2019.
41. Budsberg, S.C.; Jevens, D.J.; Brown, J.; Foutz, T.L.; DeCamp, C.E.; Reece, L. Evaluation of Limb Symmetry Indices, Using Ground Reaction Forces in Healthy Dogs. *Am. J. Vet. Res.* **1993**, *54*, 1569–1574. [CrossRef]
42. Volstad, N.J.; Sandberg, G.; Robb, S.; Budsberg, S.C. The Evaluation Of Limb Symmetry Indices Using Ground Reaction Forces Collected with One or Two Force Plates in Healthy Dogs. *Vet. Comp. Orthop. Traumatol.* **2017**, *30*, 54–58. [CrossRef]
43. Anderson, M.; Mann, F.; Wagner-Mann, C.; Hahn, A.; Jiang, B.; Tomlinson, J. A Comparison of Nonthreaded, Enhanced Threaded, and Ellis Fixation Pins Used in Type I External Skeletal Fixators in Dogs. *Vet. Surg.* **1993**, *22*, 482–489. [CrossRef]

Disclaimer/Publisher's Note: The statements, opinions and data contained in all publications are solely those of the individual author(s) and contributor(s) and not of MDPI and/or the editor(s). MDPI and/or the editor(s) disclaim responsibility for any injury to people or property resulting from any ideas, methods, instructions or products referred to in the content.

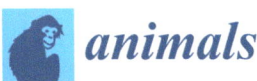

Case Report

Treatment of a Large Tibial Non-Union Bone Defect in a Cat Using Xenograft with Canine-Derived Cancellous Bone, Demineralized Bone Matrix, and Autograft

Keun-Yung Kim [1], Minha Oh [2] and Minkyung Kim [3,*]

1. Fatima Animal Medical Center, Daegu 41216, Republic of Korea
2. Veteregen, Hanam 12930, Republic of Korea
3. Keunmaum Animal Medical Center, Busan 48096, Republic of Korea
* Correspondence: vetmk@gnu.ac.kr

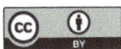

Citation: Kim, K.-Y.; Oh, M.; Kim, M. Treatment of a Large Tibial Non-Union Bone Defect in a Cat Using Xenograft with Canine-Derived Cancellous Bone, Demineralized Bone Matrix, and Autograft. *Animals* 2024, 14, 690. https://doi.org/10.3390/ani14050690

Academic Editors: L. Miguel Carreira and João Alves

Received: 10 January 2024
Revised: 16 February 2024
Accepted: 22 February 2024
Published: 22 February 2024

Copyright: © 2024 by the authors. Licensee MDPI, Basel, Switzerland. This article is an open access article distributed under the terms and conditions of the Creative Commons Attribution (CC BY) license (https://creativecommons.org/licenses/by/4.0/).

Simple Summary: In feline tibia fractures, limited tissue coverage may lead to complications such as open fractures and delayed healing. Non-union, attributed to factors such as poor blood supply, malnutrition, bone misalignment, infections, and bone damage, necessitates bone grafting for repair. While autografts are preferred, they may be insufficient for extensive defects, prompting the use of allografts and xenografts created through xenotransplantation processes such as deproteinized bovine bone. Past graft options were limited, but contemporary alternatives encompass a broader range, incorporating xenografts, demineralized bone matrix (DBM), and calcium-based materials. When combined with growth factors or cells, these materials significantly enhance their effectiveness. This case describes the treatment of a cat's tibia defect using an autologous cancellous bone graft, recombinant human bone morphogenetic protein-2, and a xenograft derived from canines mixed with DBM. Despite the initial use of external skeletal fixation and antibiotic therapy for infection, a significant defect persisted even after bone healing was complete, necessitating a multifaceted approach involving additional plate placement, autograft, and xenograft. As a result, the long-term prognosis was favorable with no complications observed in the subject's bone healing.

Abstract: A 17-month-old domestic short-hair cat was referred due to a non-union in the left tibia. The initial repair, conducted 3 months prior at another animal hospital, involved an intramedullary (IM) pin and wire to address a comminuted fracture. Unfortunately, the wire knot caused a skin tract, resulting in osteomyelitis. Although the wire knot was removed at that hospital, the draining tract persisted, continuously discharging exudate. Upon evaluation, the first surgery was reassessed and revised, involving the removal of the IM pin and the application of external skeletal fixation alongside an antibiotic susceptibility test. After 118 days post-revision surgery, while some cortical continuity was observed, a significant bone defect persisted, posing a substantial risk of refracture should the implant be removed. A second revision surgery was performed, utilizing a bone plate combined with cancellous bone autograft, recombinant human bone morphogenetic protein-2, and xenograft featuring a canine-derived cancellous chip mixed with demineralized bone matrix. Remarkably, the bone completed its healing within 105 days following the subsequent surgery. Radiography demonstrated successful management of the large bone defect up to the 2-year postoperative check-up. During telephone follow-ups for 3.5 years after surgery, no complications were identified, and the subject maintained a favorable gait.

Keywords: cats; demineralized bone matrix; large bone defect; non-union; osteomyelitis; xenograft

1. Introduction

The tibia ranks as the most frequent fracture site in cats, comprising 18.0% of all fractures, and notably contributing to 61.1% of reported non-union cases [1]. The limited soft tissue coverage along the tibia's medial surface increases the risk of complications, including open fractures, periosteal stripping, and delayed bone revascularization during the healing phase [2–4].

The etiology of non-union may involve multiple factors. A poor blood supply to the affected area, coupled with a suboptimal nutritional status, can predispose to non-union fractures [5,6]. Poor apposition of the fractured bone ends, pathological fractures, large quantities of necrotic bone, or infections have also been reported as potential etiological factors [6]. Bone grafts play a crucial role in improving healing in delayed unions, non-unions, osteotomies, arthrodesis, and multi-fragmentary fractures, as well as in replacing bony loss [7–10]. While autografts traditionally prove effective in repairing defects caused by comminuted fractures and non-unions, offering necessary mechanical stability, their application becomes challenging when dealing with extensive defects due to the limited availability of bone [11–13]. This limitation encourages exploring the use of allografts and xenografts as substitutes [14].

Xenotransplantation, involving the intentional transfer of living cells, tissues, or organs from one species to another, results in the creation of xenografts [15]. The most extensively researched and commonly employed xenograft material is deproteinized and heat-treated bovine bone [16–20]. Recently, canine-derived allografts with demineralized bone matrix (DBM) products have been developed, and related research on their application has been published [21–23]. However, comprehensive studies on the healing of bony defects in cats using canine-derived xenografts have not been fully evaluated. This case report aims to present the healing of a feline tibia with large defects after revision surgery using autologous cancellous bone grafts, recombinant human bone morphogenetic protein (BMP)-2 (rh-BMP2), and xenografts with canine-derived cancellous chips mixed with DBM.

2. Case Presentation

2.1. History and Clinical Examination

A 17-month-old, 4.91 kg, castrated male domestic short-haired cat presented with a 3-month history of non-weight-bearing lameness in the left hindlimb. The subject had sustained a fracture in an accident 3 months prior and had subsequently undergone treatment involving intramedullary (IM) pinning and wiring at a different hospital. However, complications arose as the knot on the wire became abscessed, necessitating its removal, leaving only the IM pin in place. Upon arrival at our facility, the left tibia exhibited palpable crepitus, and evident signs of inflammation, including edema, redness, warmth, and pain, were observed. Additionally, a suppurative exudate was evident through the skin tract (Figure 1A). However, the patient had not received any prescribed medications, including antibiotics, at the previous hospital, with only chlorhexidine being used for skin disinfection.

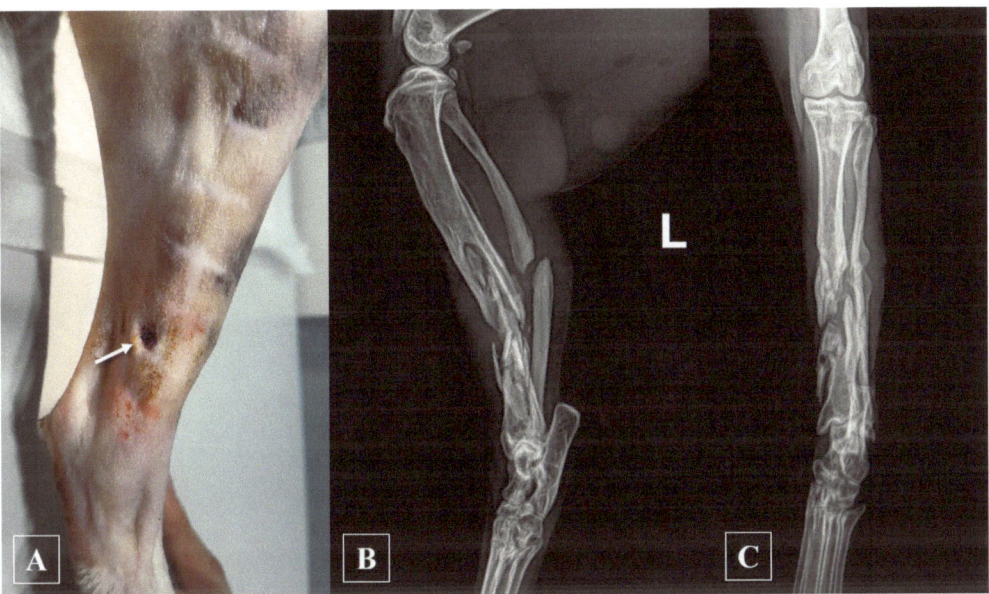

Figure 1. The appearance of the subject during the initial visit and subsequent radiographs following the removal of the intramedullary pin. (**A**) Following clipping, a skin tract and suture knot were observed on the medial side of the subject's tibia, which was accompanied by exudate discharge (arrow). A sample was collected from this area and sent for antibiotic susceptibility testing. (**B**) Mediolateral and (**C**) craniocaudal radiographs of left tibia. (L: left).

2.2. Anesthesia and Surgical Treatment

The subject's pre-anesthesia examinations, including blood work and thoracic radiography before surgery, were unremarkable. Before IM pin removal, a sample for antibiotic susceptibility testing was taken from the skin tract, and the infection site was thoroughly irrigated with normal saline until it appeared pale. Preoperative medication included prophylactic cefazolin (25 mg/kg IV; Cefazolin injection 1 g, Chongkundang, Seoul, Republic of Korea) and premedication with acepromazine (0.03 mg/kg IV; Sedaject injection, Samu median, Yesan, Republic of Korea), and ketamine (5 mg/kg IV; Ketamine HCl injection, Huons, Seongnam, Republic of Korea). General anesthesia induction employed propofol (6 mg/kg IV; Provive injection 1%, Phambio Korea, Seoul, Republic of Korea), and maintenance was carried out with isoflurane (Ifran liq., Hana Pharm, Seoul, Republic of Korea) inhalation anesthesia at an oxygen flow rate of 2 L/min. The proximal part of the IM pin was observed to protrude into the stifle joint and was therefore excised aseptically through a stab incision, employing a combination of chlorhexidine gluconate and alcohol for skin asepsis. Subsequent radiographic examination revealed a non-union in the mid-diaphysis of the left tibia (Figure 1B,C). For external skeletal fixation, the subject, positioned in left recumbency, underwent aseptic surgery. Utilizing fluoroscopy, external skeletal fixation was placed using a 2.0 mm positive threaded pin. The proximal tibial fragment was stabilized in a type 1a configuration, while the distal fragment was secured in a type 1b configuration. The pin ends were appropriately bent to align parallel to each other and then secured with wire before being further reinforced with epoxy putty (Figure 2A).

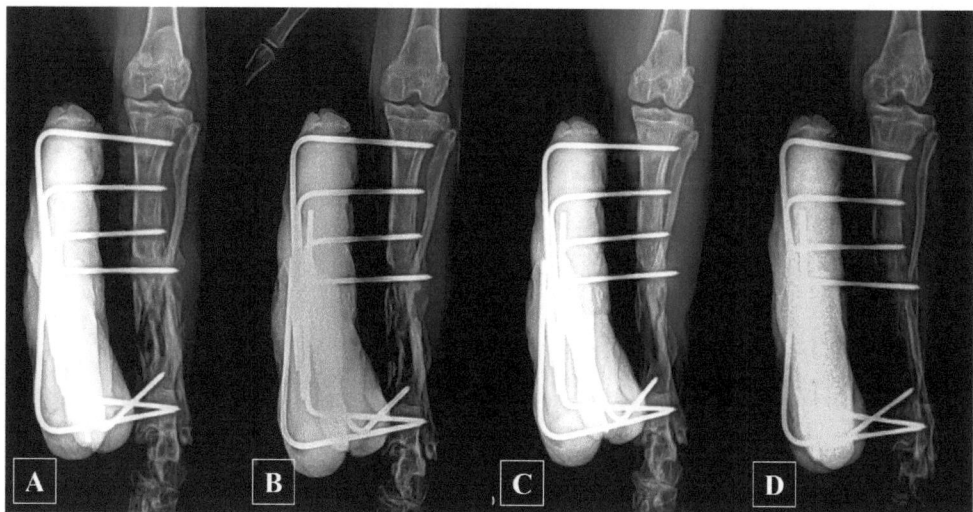

Figure 2. Craniocaudal postoperative radiographs of the left tibia depicting the utilization of external skeletal fixation with 2.0 mm positive thread pins and epoxy putty. (**A**) Immediately after surgery; (**B**) 14 days post-surgery; (**C**) 56 days post-surgery; and (**D**) 118 days post-surgery.

2.3. Postoperative Management and Prognosis

After the surgery, the subject remained in the hospital for 2 weeks. By the third postoperative day, the subject initiated small steps, progressing to a gradual improvement in gait, eventually resulting in discharge from the hospital with restored normal ambulation. Following the revision surgery, the patient received cefazolin at a dosage of 25 mg/kg intravenously twice a day (BID), famotidine at 0.5 mg/kg intravenously BID, tramadol at 2 mg/kg intravenously BID, and meloxicam at 0.3 mg/kg subcutaneously as a single shot, along with once-daily dressing changes. On the fifth day post-revision surgery, antibiotic susceptibility testing revealed cephalosporin resistance, prompting a change in antibiotic therapy. The antibiotic susceptibility test confirmed *Enterococcus* spp., resistant to various antibiotics, but susceptible to amoxicillin–clavulanate (AMC). Consequently, the subject received a 1-month course of AMC (12.5 mg/kg PO, twice a day; Amocla Tab. 375 mg, Kuhnil, Seoul, Republic of Korea) with a gastric protectant in addition to the treatment.

The exudation from the tibia ceased a week after the revision surgery, and the infection was successfully resolved with complete wound healing observed at 10 days after the revision surgery; however, the bone gradually became more osteolytic without forming a callus (Figure 2B–D). Ultimately, while some cortical continuity was observed in the caudo-lateral aspect of the tibia, a substantial defect remained in the cranio-medial aspect of the tibia, and the potential for re-fracture was deemed significantly high if the external fixator were to be removed. Consequently, a decision was made, following the evaluation of 118-day post-operative radiographs, to remove the external fixator and address the defect by filling it with bone substitutes, which was accompanied by additional fixation utilizing a plate.

The patient was anesthetized and prepped in the same manner as for the initial revision surgery. During the medial approach of the tibia, a closed IM cavity was observed (Figure 3A). The inactive bone margin was debrided using a burr and rongeur, which was followed by rimming the bone marrow cavity with a drill bit to ensure better visibility of blood flow (Figure 3B,C). All procedures were conducted with chilled saline to prevent thermal damage and aimed to minimize bone loss. Subsequently, the tibia was stabilized using a 1.5/2.0 mm locking compression plate (DePuy Synthes Vet, Solothurn, Switzerland) positioned on the medial surface and secured with 2.0 mm locking screws. Three screws were inserted into the proximal bone fragment, and two screws were placed in the distal bone fragment. Following the application of plates and screws, autologous cancellous bone was aseptically harvested from the left humeral head. This bone was then combined with synthetic substitutes, cancellous bone derived from canines mixed with DBM (NatraOss; Veteregen, Hanam, Republic of Korea), along with rh-BMP2 (Novosis; CGBIO, Seoul, Republic of Korea). The bone graft mixture was meticulously applied to fill the large defect beneath the plate, and the skin was closed routinely (Figure 3D). The subject exhibited good mobility both before and after the surgery, prompting their discharge home on the third day post-operation.

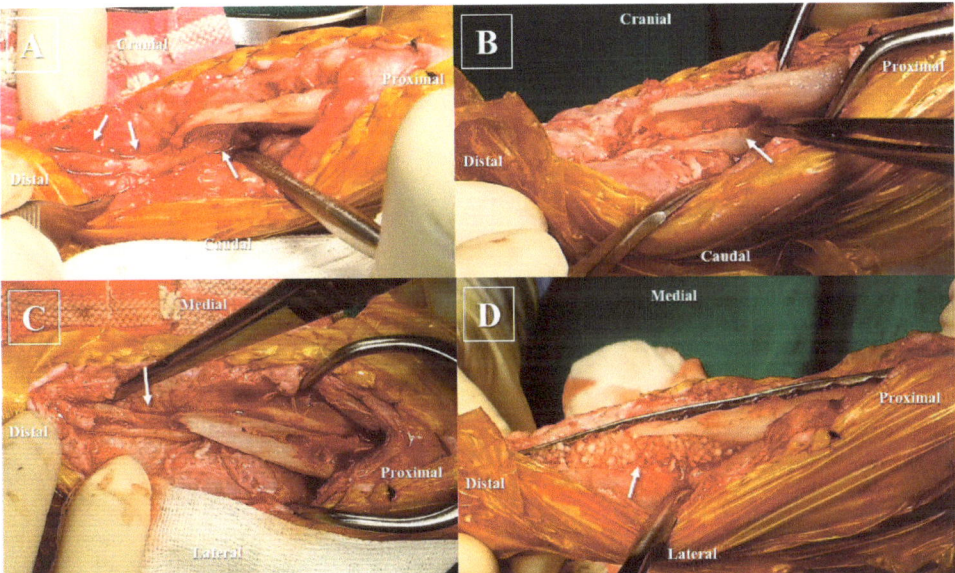

Figure 3. Intraoperative photos illustrating the subject's procedure. (**A**) Immediately after soft tissue separation, significant defects and obstructed medullary cavities were revealed (arrows); (**B**) the final size of the proximal defect is shown in the lateral view (arrow). The proximal bone margin underwent decortication and was rimmed with a burr, rongeur, and drill-bit; (**C**) craniocaudal perspective displaying the distal bone after decortication, indicating visible blood supply from the bone (arrow); (**D**) application of bone substitutes to fill the defect after plate application (arrow). This included a mixture of autologous cancellous bone, recombinant human bone morphogenetic protein-2, and a canine-derived cancellous chip mixed with demineralized bone matrix.

At 28 days after the second revision surgery, the radiographic examination revealed cortical bridging, and the bone graft exhibited signs of resorption, although some areas remained unbridged (Figure 4B). However, by the 105-day mark post-surgery, a subsequent check confirmed complete cortical bridging across all areas, which was accompanied by bone remodeling (Figure 4C). At the 2-year postoperative follow-up, the subject exhibited an uneventful physical exam, a normal gait, and radiographic evidence indicating further cortical bone remodeling and reshaping compared to the previous assessment at the graft site (Figure 4D). Subsequently, phone follow-ups regarding the subject were undertaken until 3.5 years post-surgery, confirming normal walking ability and the absence of any complications.

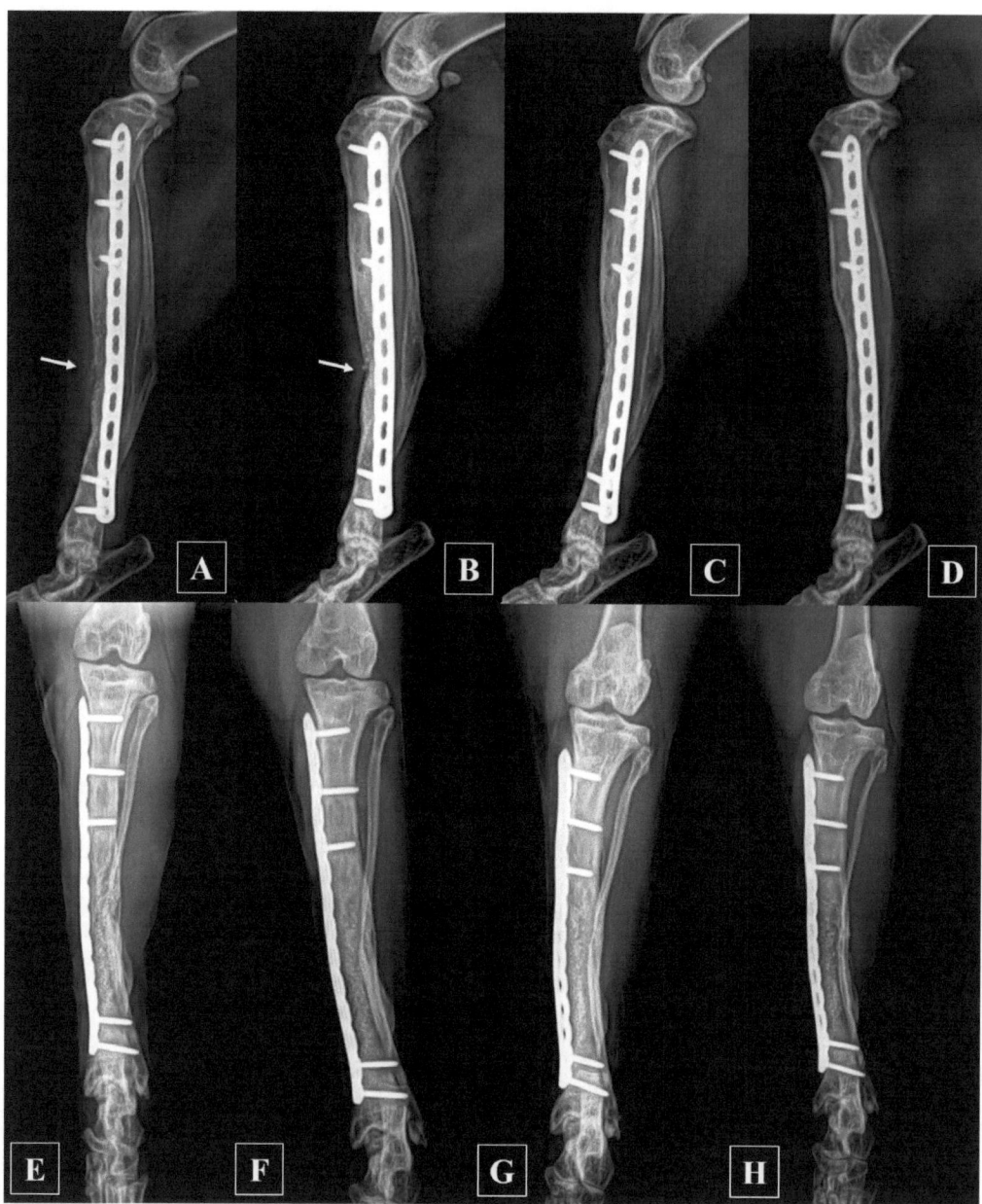

Figure 4. Mediolateral postoperative radiographs of the left tibia were taken with slight internal rotation to assess the plate-concealed bone area. (**A**) At 7 days after surgery, there was no bridging of the cortex observed, and the bone substitutes remained visible (arrow); (**B**) at 28 days after surgery, the bridging of the cortex was confirmed; however, there was still no continuity observed in certain areas (arrow); (**C**) at 105 days post-surgery, bridging of the cortex was observed in all sections; (**D**) two years post-surgery, further bone remodeling occurred, enhancing the distinction between cortical and cancellous bone. Craniocaudal postoperative radiographs of the left tibia: (**E**) immediately after surgery; (**F**) 42 days post-surgery; (**G**) 105 days post-surgery; (**H**) two years post-surgery.

3. Discussion

Fracture healing necessitates osteogenic cells, an osteoconductive matrix, an osteoinductive stimulus, mechanical stability, and adequate vascular supply [24]. Deficiency in any of these elements can lead to delayed union or non-union, with non-union fractures developing under various circumstances, including inadequate fixation, compromised blood supply, infection, presence of soft tissue between fragments, or substantial gaps between fracture fragments [1,25,26]. In our subject's case, osteomyelitis and insufficient mechanical stability due to inadequate implant selection (IM pin and wire) led to non-union at presentation. Additionally, the distal location of the fracture in the tibia, commonly associated with longer healing durations compared to proximal long bones, could be attributed to diminished soft tissue coverage and a relatively poorer blood supply [1]. To address these issues, we implemented external skeletal fixation and antibiotic therapy to treat the infection, which was followed by the restoration of the bone defect using a xenograft along with bone plate application.

External skeletal fixation was chosen as the primary method to address the infection due to concerns that plates might exacerbate it by extending the affected area. Additionally, suspected low bone density resulting from the infection and lack of use necessitated the need for bone stabilization. The external skeletal fixator can be removed once clinical union, defined as the presence of a bridging callus on three of four cortices on two orthogonal radiographic views, has been reached [27]. However, in our case, even though the surgical site infection was effectively treated and confirmed partial bone healing following the initial revision surgery, the substantial defect within the bone created a high likelihood of bone re-fracture if the implant was to be removed. Hence, our strategy entailed addressing the bone defect by employing bone graft material and reinforcing stabilization with an additional plate fixation.

Segmental cortical defects averaging 1.5 times the bone diaphyseal diameter are known to impair bone healing in dogs and cats [26]. Enhanced bone regeneration is justified in cases of non-union not only to provide support and fill existing lacunae but also to enhance biological repair when the skeletal defect reaches the so-called critical size [28]. Over the years, the use of bone substitute materials has traditionally been limited to cancellous and cortical autografts or allografts; however, modern alternatives now encompass a range of bone graft substitutes, including xenografts, DBM, and calcium-based materials. Ongoing research explores the incorporation of growth factors, osteoprogenitor cells, or both, in combination with bone grafts or graft substitutes [29]. The final selection of which bone substitute material to use is subsequently based on the specific requirements of the actual clinical situation [30].

In our subject, the limited availability of cancellous bone autograft compared to the defect size prompted the exploration of additional methods to comprehensively address the issue. To address this clinical situation, we adopted a product combining canine-derived cancellous bony chips with DBM as a xenograft and rh-BMP2, alongside cancellous bone autograft, aiming to increase the engraftment success rate for this subject [31]. Although xenografts are convenient for storage and use, they possess considerably less capacity for osteoinduction and osteoconduction compared to autografts [14]. To address the shortcomings of these xenografts, additional materials, such as rh-BMP2 and cancellous bone autograft, have been incorporated.

The incorporation of cancellous bone xenografts combined with DBM, derived through the decalcification of cortical bone, significantly enhances osteoinductive properties. This process reduces mineral content, enhancing graft flexibility for precise placement. Moreover, combining DBM with adjuncts like hydroxyapatite, autografts, or bone marrow aspirate further refines its manipulative qualities and mechanical strength. Consequently, we integrated it with a small quantity of autograft harvested from the humeral head [20,32].

Furthermore, the integration of BMPs was employed to bolster osteoinductive capabilities. BMPs serve as differentiation factors, which are primarily responsible for prompting the transformation of undifferentiated mesenchymal cells into chondroblasts [33]. It was suggested that BMP2, BMP6, and BMP9 may play an important role in inducing the osteoblast differentiation of mesenchymal stem cells, whereas, in contrast, most BMPs are able to stimulate osteogenesis in mature osteoblasts [34]. Recent recombinant technology has allowed the isolation, production, and application of these synthesized molecules for osteoinductive and osteoconductive purposes required for healing bone defects [35]. Interspecies amino acid sequence homology for rh-BMP2 is 100% in most mammalian species, thus allowing for its use in all species that are commonly treated by veterinary fields [14].

The most commonly used xenograft is bovine-derived, and there have been several successful applications in humans, dogs, and cats [16,36,37]. Xenografts demonstrate promise; however, it is essential to take into account the possibility of immune rejection, which has been primarily attributed to the presence of a cell and matrix surface carbohydrate antigen known as the α-galactosyl epitope [38]. The presence of foreign material can trigger an antigenic response, heightening the risk of graft rejection, with a greater likelihood of rejection observed when utilizing pure bone xenografts [14]. To address these issues, the process for bovine-derived cancellous bone material involves boiling, defatting, and deproteination while aiming to preserve the stiffness, internal structure, and minimize immune responses [39].

Recent reports have documented successful applications of allografts in dogs, but using dog-derived bone grafts in cats remains undocumented [22]. Foreseeing decreased complications owing to the xenograft's pre-processing and anticipating diminished immune reactivity in our subjects, the adoption of a canine-derived xenograft was contemplated to potentially aid the bone-healing mechanism, leading to its selection for our subject's treatment.

This report represents the first instance, to the authors' knowledge, of using a canine-derived xenograft to address non-union in a cat. Nevertheless, certain limitations exist within this case report. Firstly, due to its nature as a case report rather than a research study, objective comparisons with other established grafts for effectiveness were not feasible. Secondly, during the initial 2 years, the subject underwent radiographic follow-ups; however, subsequent monitoring has solely relied on phone follow-ups. While the subject's gait remains favorable, conducting longer-term bone assessments has not been feasible, posing limitations in tracking bone status over time. Despite some limitations, this case demonstrated successful bone union and regained normal gait without complications. The use of canine-derived xenografts, similar to conventional bovine-derived xenografts, presents promising advantages in addressing significant non-union bone defects in cats, particularly when applied alongside autologous bone and various other bone graft substitutes to enhance outcomes.

4. Conclusions

In cases of significant bone defects resulting from non-union, exclusive reliance on autografts may be insufficient, prompting the need for alternative approaches. Our subject exhibited positive outcomes following treatment with a canine-derived xenograft, akin to the commonly used bovine-derived xenograft, complemented by autograft and rhBMP-2 to mitigate xenograft limitations [20]. This combined therapeutic regimen resulted in the subject's successful recovery devoid of complications, indicating the potential efficacy of canine-derived xenografts as a viable treatment option for feline subjects managing substantial bone defects.

Author Contributions: Conceptualization, K.-Y.K. and M.O.; methodology, K.-Y.K.; investigation, M.O.; writing—original draft preparation, K.-Y.K.; writing—review and editing, M.K.; supervision, M.K. All authors have read and agreed to the published version of the manuscript.

Funding: This research received no external funding.

Institutional Review Board Statement: The cat was treated according to its clinical symptoms, and the clinical procedures involving the animal were carried out in accordance with biosafety and ethical guidelines.

Informed Consent Statement: Informed consent was obtained from the owner of the subject cat.

Data Availability Statement: The data presented in this study are available on request from the corresponding author. The data are not publicly available due to privacy or ethical restrictions.

Conflicts of Interest: Minha Oh is an employee of Veteregen; however, this research was not funded by the company nor did it receive any financial support or benefits from Veteregen.

References

1. Nolte, D.M.; Fusco, V.F.; Peterson, M.E. Incidence of and predisposing factors for non union of fractures involving the appendicular skeleton in cats. *J. Am. Vet. Med. Assoc.* **2005**, *226*, 77–82. [CrossRef] [PubMed]
2. Richardson, E.F.; Thacher, C.W. Tibial fractures in cats. *Compend. Cont. Educ.* **1993**, *15*, 383–393.
3. Boone, E.G.; Johnson, A.L.; Montavon, P.; Hohn, R.B. Fractures of the tibial diaphysis in dogs and cats. *J. Am. Vet. Med. Assoc.* **1986**, *188*, 41–45. [PubMed]
4. Harari, J. Treatments for feline long bone fractures. *Vet. Clin. North Am. Small Anim. Pract.* **2002**, *32*, 927–947. [CrossRef] [PubMed]
5. Dugat, D.; Rochat, M.; Ritchey, J.; Payton, M. Quantitative analysis of the intramedullary arterial supply of the feline tibia. *Vet. Comp. Orthop. Traumatol.* **2011**, *24*, 313–319. [CrossRef]
6. Stevens, A.; Lowe, J.S. *Pathology*, 1st ed.; Elsevier Health Sciences: Philadelphia, PA, USA, 1995.
7. Alexander, J.W. Bone grafting. *Vet. Clin. North Am. Small Anim. Pract.* **1987**, *17*, 811–819. [CrossRef] [PubMed]
8. Alexander, J.W. Bone grafting. In *Leonard's Orthopaedic Surgery of the Dog and Cat*, 3rd ed.; Alexander, J.W., Ed.; WB Saunders: Philadelphia, PA, USA, 1985; pp. 43–48.
9. Brinker, W.O.; Piermattei, D.L.; Flo, G.L. Bone grafting. In *Small Animal Orthopaedics and Fracture Repair*, 3rd ed.; Piermattei, D.L., Ed.; WB Saunders: Philadelphia, PA, USA, 1997; pp. 147–153. [CrossRef]
10. Fox, S.M. Cancellous bone grafting in the dog: An overview. *J. Am. Anim. Hosp. Assoc.* **1984**, *20*, 840–848.
11. Dorea, H.C.; McLaughlin, R.M.; Cantwell, H.D.; Read, R.; Armbrust, L.; Pool, R.; Roush, J.K.; Boyle, C. Evaluation of healing in feline femoral defects filled with cancellous autograft, cancellous allograft or Bioglass. *Vet. Comp. Orthop. Traumatol.* **2005**, *18*, 157–168. [CrossRef]
12. Kerwin, S.C.; Lewis, D.D.; Elkins, A.D. Bone grafting and banking. *Compend. Contin. Educ. Vet.* **1991**, *13*, 1558–1566.
13. Sinibaldi, K.R. Evaluation of full cortical allografts in 25 dogs. *J. Am. Vet Medic Assoc.* **1989**, *194*, 1570–1577.
14. Vertenten, G.; Gasthuys, F.; Cornelissen, M.; Schacht, E.; Vlaminck, L. Enhancing bone healing and regeneration: Present and future perspectives in veterinary orthopaedics. *Vet. Comp. Orthop. Traumatol.* **2010**, *23*, 153–162. [CrossRef]
15. Snell, G.D. The terminology of tissue transplantation. *Transplantation* **1964**, *2*, 655–657.
16. Tuominen, T.; Jamsa, T.; Tuukkanen, J.; Marttinen, A.; Lindholm, T.S.; Jalovaara, P. Bovine bone implant with bovine bone morphogenetic protein in healing a canine ulnar defect. *Int. Orthop.* **2001**, *25*, 5–8. [CrossRef]
17. Young, C.; Sandstedt, P.; Skoglund, A. A comparative study of anorganic xenogenic bone and autogenous bone implants for bone regeneration in rabbits. *Int. J. Oral. Maxillofac. Implant.* **1999**, *14*, 72–76.
18. Hollinger, J.O.; Schmitz, J.P.; Mark, D.E.; Seyfer, A.E. Osseous wound healing with xenogeneic bone implants with a biodegradable carrier. *Surgery* **1990**, *107*, 50–54.
19. Worth, A.J.; Thompson, K.G.; Owen, M.C.; Mucalo, M.R.; Firth, E.C. Combined xeno/auto-grafting of a benign osteolytic lesion in a dog, using a novel bovine cancellous bone biomaterial. *New Zealand Vet. J.* **2007**, *55*, 143–148. [CrossRef]
20. Kao, S.T.; Scott, D.D. A review of bone substitutes. *Oral. Maxillofac. Surg. Clin. North Am.* **2007**, *19*, 513–521. [CrossRef]
21. Hoffer, M.J.; Griffon, D.J.; Schaeffer, D.J.; Johnson, A.L.; Thomas, M.W. Clinical applications of demineralized bone matrix: A retrospective and case-matched study of seventy-five dogs. *Vet. Surg.* **2008**, *37*, 639–647. [CrossRef] [PubMed]
22. Lafaver, S.; Miller, N.A.; Stubbs, W.P.; Taylor, R.A.; Boudrieau, R.J. Tibial tuberosity advancement for stabilization of the canine cranial cruciate ligament-deficient stifle joint: Surgical technique, early results, and complications in 101 dogs. *Vet. Surg.* **2007**, *36*, 573–586. [CrossRef] [PubMed]
23. Innes, J.F.; Myint, P. Demineralised bone matrix in veterinary orthopaedics: A review. *Vet Comp. Orthop. Traumatol.* **2010**, *23*, 393–399. [CrossRef] [PubMed]
24. Calori, G.M.; Giannoudis, P.V. Enhancement of fracture healing with the diamond concept: The role of the biological chamber. *Injury* **2011**, *42*, 1191–1193. [CrossRef]
25. Key, J.A. The effect of a local calcium depot on osteogenesis and healing of fractures. *J. Bone Joint. Surg.* **1934**, *16A*, 176–184.
26. Toombs, J.P.; Wallace, L.J.; Bjorling, D.E.; Rowland, G.N. Evaluation of Key's hypothesis in the feline tibia: An experimental model for augmented bone healing studies. *Am. J. Vet. Res.* **1985**, *46*, 513–518. [PubMed]
27. DeCamp, C.E.; Johnson, S.A.; Schaefer, S.L. *Brinker, Piermattei, and Flo's Handbook of Small Anim.al Orthopedics and Fracture Repair*, 5th ed.; Saunders: Philadelphia, PA, USA, 2016; pp. 674–679.
28. Olivier, V.; Faucheux, N.; Hardouin, P. Biomaterial challenges and approaches to stem cell use in bone reconstructive surgery. *Drug Discov. Today* **2004**, *9*, 803–811. [CrossRef]
29. Kolk, A.; Handschel, J.; Drescher, W.; Rothamel, D.; Kloss, F.; Blessmann, M.; Heiland, M.; Wolff, K.D.; Smeets, R. Current trends and future perspectives of bone substitute materials—From space holders to innovative biomaterials. *J. Craniomaxillofac. Surg.* **2012**, *40*, 706–718. [CrossRef] [PubMed]

30. Millis, D.L.; Martinez, S.A. Bone grafts. In *Textbook of Small Animal Surgery*, 3rd ed.; Slatter, D., Ed.; WB Saunders Company: Philadelphia, PA, USA, 2003; Volume 2, pp. 1875–1891.
31. Bharadwaz, A.; Jayasuriya, A.C. Osteogenic differentiation cues of the bone morphogenetic protein-9 (BMP-9) and its recent advances in bone tissue regeneration. *Mater. Sci. Eng. C* **2021**, *120*, 111748. [CrossRef]
32. Mahendra, A.; Maclean, A.D. Available biological treatments for complex non-unions. *Injury* **2007**, *38*, S7–S12. [CrossRef]
33. Kirker-Head, C.A. Recombinant bone morphogenetic proteins: Novel substances for enhancing bone healing. *Vet. Surg.* **1995**, *24*, 408–419. [CrossRef]
34. Cheng, H.; Jiang, W.; Phillips, F.M.; Haydon, R.C.; Peng, Y.; Zhou, L.; Luu, H.H.; An, N.; Breyer, B.; Vanichakarn, P.; et al. Osteogenic activity of the fourteen types of human bone morphogenetic proteins (BMPs). *J. Bone Jt. Surg. Am.* **2003**, *85*, 1544–1552. [CrossRef] [PubMed]
35. Simpson, A.H.; Mills, L.; Noble, B. The role of growth factors and related agents in accelerating fracture healing. *J. Bone Jt. Surg. Br.* **2006**, *88*, 701–705. [CrossRef]
36. Bansal, M.R.; Bhagat, S.B.; Shukla, D.D. Bovine cancellous xenograft in the treatment of tibial plateau fractures in elderly patients. *Int. Orthop.* **2009**, *33*, 779–784. [CrossRef]
37. Dulaurent, T.; Azoulay, T.; Goulle, F.; Dulaurent, A.; Mentek, M.; Peiffer, R.L.; Isard, P.F. Use of bovine pericardium (Tutopatch(R)) graft for surgical repair of deep melting corneal ulcers in dogs and corneal sequestra in cats. *Vet. Ophthalmol.* **2014**, *17*, 91–99. [CrossRef] [PubMed]
38. Na, J.Y.; Song, K.; Kim, S.; Lee, H.B.; Kim, J.K.; Kim, J.H.; Lee, J.W.; Kwon, J. Evaluation of porcine xenograft in collateral ligament reconstruction in beagle dogs. *Res. Vet. Sci.* **2014**, *97*, 605–610. [CrossRef] [PubMed]
39. Anderson, I.A.; Mucalo, M.R.; Johnson, G.S.; Lorier, M.A. The processing and characterization of animal-derived bone to yield materials with biomedical applications. Part III: Material and mechanical properties of fresh and processed bovine cancellous bone. *J. Mater. Sci. Mater. Med.* **2000**, *11*, 743–749. [CrossRef] [PubMed]

Disclaimer/Publisher's Note: The statements, opinions and data contained in all publications are solely those of the individual author(s) and contributor(s) and not of MDPI and/or the editor(s). MDPI and/or the editor(s) disclaim responsibility for any injury to people or property resulting from any ideas, methods, instructions or products referred to in the content.

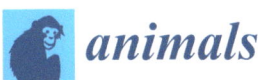

Article

Assessing the Effectiveness of Modified Tibial Plateau Leveling Osteotomy Plates for Treating Cranial Cruciate Ligament Rupture and Medial Patellar Luxation in Small-Breed Dogs

Eunbin Jeong [1,†], Youngjin Jeon [2,†], Taewan Kim [1], Dongbin Lee [1] and Yoonho Roh [1,*]

1 Department of Veterinary Surgery, College of Veterinary Medicine, Gyeongsang National University, Jinju 52828, Republic of Korea; dmsqls1196@gmail.com (E.J.); abcball@naver.com (T.K.); dlee@gnu.ac.kr (D.L.)
2 Department of Veterinary Surgery, College of Veterinary Medicine, Chungnam National University, Daejeon 34134, Republic of Korea; orangee0115@gmail.com
* Correspondence: yoonhoroh@gnu.ac.kr
† These authors contributed equally to this work.

Simple Summary: In small-breed dogs, medial patellar luxation and cranial cruciate ligament rupture often occur concurrently in the adult dog, presenting through diverse mechanisms. Numerous methods have been developed to treat these conditions together. The combined osteotomy method may elevate the risk of joint instability and fractures. Therefore, a pre-contoured modified tibial plateau leveling osteotomy plate was designed to achieve the dual effect of tibial tuberosity transposition, a surgery performed in kneecap dislocation correction, alongside reducing the tibial plateau angle. In this cadaveric study, we examined the efficacy and stability of this modified plate. The findings indicate that this pre-contoured plate effectively prevents forward displacement of the tibia (shinbone) and medial (inner) dislocation of the kneecap while maintaining stability.

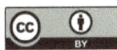

Citation: Jeong, E.; Jeon, Y.; Kim, T.; Lee, D.; Roh, Y. Assessing the Effectiveness of Modified Tibial Plateau Leveling Osteotomy Plates for Treating Cranial Cruciate Ligament Rupture and Medial Patellar Luxation in Small-Breed Dogs. *Animals* **2024**, *14*, 1937. https://doi.org/10.3390/ani14131937

Academic Editors: L. Miguel Carreira and João Alves

Received: 10 June 2024
Revised: 24 June 2024
Accepted: 29 June 2024
Published: 30 June 2024

Copyright: © 2024 by the authors. Licensee MDPI, Basel, Switzerland. This article is an open access article distributed under the terms and conditions of the Creative Commons Attribution (CC BY) license (https:// creativecommons.org/licenses/by/ 4.0/).

Abstract: In small-breed dogs with concurrent cranial cruciate ligament rupture (CCLR) and medial patellar luxation (MPL), correcting both disorders is are essential for restoring normal gait. However, the previously described surgical treatment, using two osteotomy technique, poses a high risk of fracture and instability. Addressing CCLR and MPL with a single osteotomy and implant was considered superior to the conventional method. Therefore, a pre-contoured modified tibial plateau leveling osteotomy (PCM–TPLO) plate facilitating medial shifting of the proximal tibia was developed. We compared postoperative alignment and strength between this novel plate group and a conventional tibial plateau leveling osteotomy (TPLO) plate group using eight small-breed dog cadavers each. Additionally, we investigated the potential of the novel plate as an alternative to tibial tuberosity transposition. Postoperative alignment and strength were assessed through radiographs and mechanical testing. Measurements including tibial plateau angle, mechanical medial proximal tibial angle, and number of screws within the joint were also analyzed. There were no significant differences in all measured parameters. For the novel plate, the medial displacement ratio of the proximal tibia was confirmed to be approximately 30%, and the result was thought to be appropriate. These findings suggest that the PCM–TPLO plate could be a promising alternative for treating concurrent CCLR and MPL in small-breed dogs.

Keywords: cranial cruciate ligament rupture; medial patellar luxation; tibial plateau leveling osteotomy; tibial tuberosity transposition; modified tibial plateau leveling osteotomy; dogs

1. Introduction

Cranial cruciate ligament rupture (CCLR) and medial patellar luxation (MPL) are widely recognized as prevalent causes of hindlimb lameness in dogs [1,2]. While MPL and CCLR can manifest independently, their concurrent occurrence has been observed in 6–25% of cases in small-breed dogs, with older dogs being more susceptible [3–6]. Although the exact etiology of concurrent MPL and CCLR remains unclear, a wide range of anatomical and biomechanical factors are considered to play a role in their occurrence [1,4,7]. The pathogenesis of MPL is often characterized by an aberrant arrangement of the muscles responsible for the quadriceps mechanism and bone deformities of the femur and tibia, leading to persistent joint instability and abnormal tibial movement [8,9]. This, in turn, may culminate in increased stress on the ligaments, potentially resulting in cruciate ligament tears and laxity [4,10,11]. Conversely, partial damage to the cruciate ligament, resulting in joint instability, may induce joint laxity and subsequently contribute to the development of MPL [3]. A thorough understanding of the onset and impact of these diseases is crucial for effective surgical intervention [12].

Various surgical procedures have been developed for dogs with concurrent MPL and CCLR [12–15]. Among these, the tibial plateau leveling osteotomy (TPLO) procedure is widely used for treating CCLR [13,16]. Initially introduced by Slocum in 1993, TPLO involves making a circular osteotomy in the proximal portion of the tibia and rotating it to reduce the angle of the tibial plateau, thereby alleviating cranial tibial thrust [12,17]. To correct MPL, procedures such as trochleoplasty and tibial tuberosity transposition (TTT) are commonly used [13,18]. These methods aim to reposition the patella and stabilize the extensor mechanism. TTT, a significant component of MPL surgery, involves making a partial osteotomy of the proximal tibial tuberosity and lateral repositioning of this [13]. These surgical interventions significantly alleviate lameness associated with MPL and CCLR [12]. Combining TTT and TPLO is emerging as a preferred method for correcting both conditions simultaneously [15,16]. However, performing TPLO surgery and trochleoplasty, especially TTT, concurrently in small-breed dogs presents challenges due to anatomical constraints [12,15,16,19–21]. Limited space increases the likelihood of interference between screws and pins, often leading to improper placement of the implant and compromised stability [15,19,21]. Additionally, this procedure carries an increased risk of tibial tuberosity fracture or avulsion due to the creation of two osteotomy lines in the proximal tibia [15,19,21]. Performing these surgeries separately poses challenges due to increased risks associated with anesthesia and prolonged recovery times [12,20]. Given that these conditions typically coexist in elderly dogs [3], addressing both issues in a single surgical procedure appears reasonable [12,14,15,22,23].

To mitigate these risks, modified TPLO surgical techniques have been developed to reduce costs and minimize the risks associated with anesthesia in multiple procedures [12,14,15,19–21]. This modification involves adapting the standard TPLO plate to enable medial shifting fixation of the proximal tibia, potentially combining the benefits of both TPLO and TTT procedures [12,14,15,22]. However, the process of contouring the plate during surgery may prolong operation time and result in varied outcomes depending on the surgeon's experience [14]. To address these challenges, several pre-contoured plates and patient-specific implants using 3D printing techniques have been specifically developed for small-breed dogs [9]. During the TPLO procedure, the application of a pre-contoured plate post-osteotomy facilitates medial shifting of the proximal segment, effectively replicating the outcomes of TTT [20]. A novel design of a pre-contoured TPLO plate, angled medially by 2 mm, has been introduced for small-breed dogs, offering advantages such as reduced operation time and increased consistency between surgeons [20]. Despite these advantages, there is currently no confirmation regarding whether contouring affects plate stability and provides adequate medialization in small-breed dogs [12,14].

This study aimed to assess and confirm the efficacy of the pre-contoured modified TPLO (PCM–TPLO) plate through a comparative analysis with the traditional TPLO plate group. The study focused on evaluating bone alignment and the capacity for adequate medialization in small-breed dogs, incorporating mechanical testing to assess the stability of the interface between the bone and the plate. The underlying hypothesis suggests that the PCM–TPLO plate not only offers a feasible alternative to TTT but also ensures stability and alignment comparable to that of the traditional TPLO plate.

2. Materials and Methods

2.1. Plates

The 1.5/2.0 mm PCM–TPLO plate (Jeil Medical Corp., Seoul, Republic of Korea), made of 316 L stainless steel, was designed to improve alignment and stability in surgical repairs for small-breed dogs (Figure 1). Notably, the newly developed PCM–TPLO plate is engineered with a 2 mm medial inclination, specifically crafted to promote a 2 mm lateral shift of the distal segment upon application (Figure 1D) [24]. The three proximal holes and two distal holes are designed to be engaged with locking screws. The other hole is a dynamic compression hole, providing axial compression when used with a cortical screw.

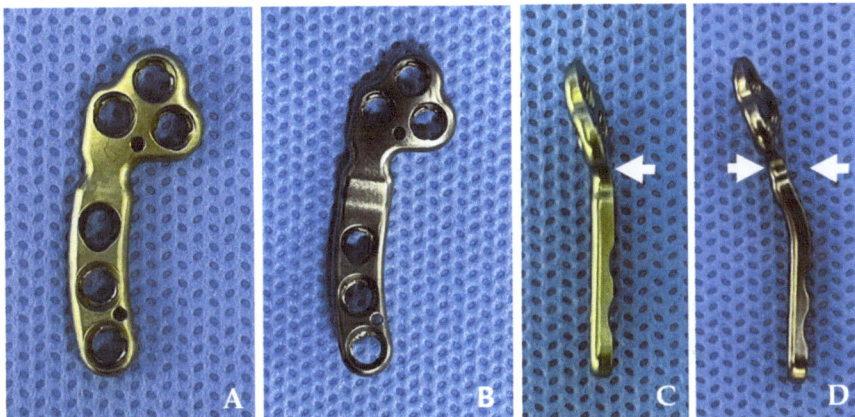

Figure 1. These figures depict a conventional tibial plateau leveling osteotomy (TPLO) plate, showing its frontal view (**A**) and side profile (**C**). The pre-contoured modified TPLO plate is presented in the frontal view (**B**) and side profile (**D**). The pre-contoured plate is specifically shaped to conform closely to the medial aspect of the tibia, intended to induce a relative medial shift of the proximal segment by 2 mm. The white arrows highlight the region of medialization.

2.2. Specimens

Sixteen stifle joints from eight small-breed dog cadavers were used in this study. All dogs were owned by clients and were euthanized for reasons unrelated to this research, then generously donated to our research team. The cadavers, each weighing between 3 and 5 kg, had no prior history of orthopedic conditions, including MPL or CCLR. A radiographic examination was conducted to confirm the absence of any anatomical abnormalities. Before the procedure, the cadavers were frozen and stored at −20 °C, then thoroughly thawed at room temperature. The 16 stifle joints were randomly divided into two groups: the conventional TPLO plate and PCM–TPLO plate groups, each comprising eight stifles. Care was taken to ensure that the stifle joints from an individual cadaver were evenly distributed between the two groups.

2.3. Surgical Procedures

Mediolateral and craniocaudal radiographs were obtained to assess the osteotomy site and identify any anatomical deformities (Figure 2). The same surgical planning approach was maintained for both groups throughout the study by a surgeon (E.B.J). The tibial plateau angle (TPA) was measured in the mediolateral view, following the method described by Slocum and Devine [25], while the mechanical medial proximal tibial angle (mMPTA) was measured in the craniocaudal view using the approach described by Dismukes et al. [26,27]. Specific measurements denoted as D1, D2, and D3 were taken to determine the osteotomy site using the standard method previously described [20].

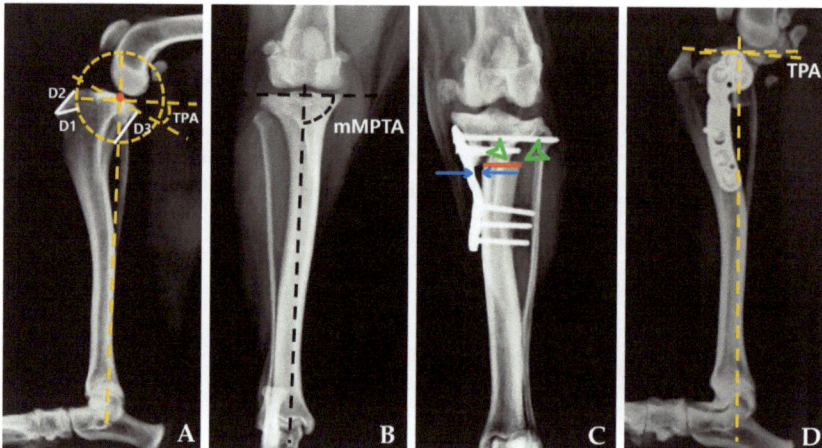

Figure 2. Pre- and postoperative mediolateral and craniocaudal radiographs for TPLO. Preoperative mediolateral radiographs illustrating measurements of the tibial plateau angle (TPA), D1 is the distance from the perpendicular cranial straight edge of the tibial crest at the most cranio-proximal point of the tibial tuberosity to the intended osteotomy site. D2 extends from the most cranio-proximal point of the tibial tuberosity to where the intended tibial osteotomy intersects the cranial tibial subchondral bone. D3 measures from the subchondral bone at the most caudal margin of the tibial plateau to where the intended tibial osteotomy intersects the caudal tibial cortex (**A**). The preoperative measurement of mMPTA is depicted in (**B**). Postoperative radiographic measurements conducted on craniocaudal radiographs for the PCM–TPLO group (**C**) include tibial osteotomy width (red line), bone–plate gap (blue arrow), and medialization distance (green arrowhead). The postoperative measurement of TPA is shown in (**D**).

All subsequent procedures were performed by a single surgeon (E.B.J) based on the earlier surgical planning. The TPLO surgery aimed to achieve a postoperative TPA of 5° [17,24]. The surgeon selected either an 8 or 10 mm saw TPLO blade depending on the size of the cadaver. In cases involving the PCM–TPLO plate, the surgery followed the same method, with an emphasis on maximizing contact between the plate and bone to displace the proximal tibial fragment medially (Figure 2C,D).

2.4. Postoperative Measurements

2.4.1. Radiographic Measurements

Following the surgical procedure, mediolateral and craniocaudal radiographs were obtained following the same protocol. Postoperative measurements, including TPA, mMPTA, the number of screws within the joint, bone–plate gap, medialization distance, and tibial osteotomy width, were then conducted based on these radiographic images and gross assessment (Figures 2 and 3). For cases involving PCM–TPLO, an assessment of the extent of medial translation was performed. This parameter was assessed as the percentage value between medialization distance and tibial osteotomy width.

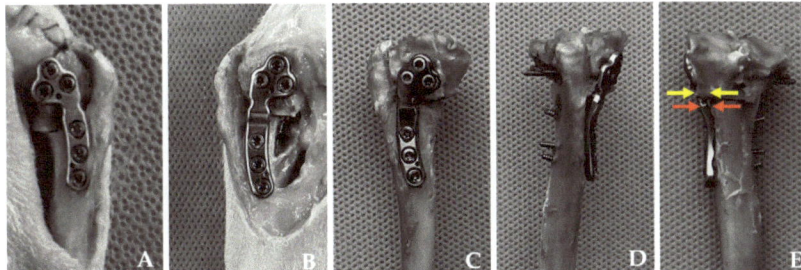

Figure 3. Intraoperative images illustrating the attachment of the TPLO plate (**A**) and the pre-contoured modified (PCM) TPLO plate (**B**) to the tibia. Measurements of the dissected tibiae of the PCM–TPLO groups (**C–E**). Medial, anterior, and posterior views after removal of soft tissues and the fibula attached to the tibia (**C–E**). The extent of medial translation of the proximal segment was measured using calipers (yellow arrows), while the gaps between the bone and plate were measured (red arrows).

2.4.2. Compression Test

Following postoperative radiography, we surgically removed all soft tissues and the fibula attached to the tibia. To prevent any interference with the compression test, a 5 mm distal section from the widest part of the tibial tuberosity was excised. An osteotomy was then performed 60 mm distal to the furthest point of the TPLO plate. The mechanical axis of the tibial bone model was aligned perpendicular to the table and securely affixed to a 3D resin jig using plaster (Mungyo Corp., Gimhae, Republic of Korea). This ensured that neither the plate nor the screws were obstructed by the plaster. Similarly, we secured the proximal part of the bone model to prevent the plate and screws from being covered by the plaster. The cadaveric specimens, integrated with the 3D resin jig made from 3D printing UV-sensitive resin (Anycubic, Shenzhen, China), were then positioned in a static load testing machine (Z010 TN; Zwick Roell, Ulm, Germany) equipped with a stainless-steel jig designed to accommodate the 3D resin jig (Figure 4). After applying a preload of 5 N, an axial compressive force was applied at a rate of 2 mm/min until implant failure occurred [28]. Standard force–time curves were generated under these test conditions, with implant failure being defined as the maximum load immediately before a sudden decrease in the continuously applied load [29].

2.5. Statistical Analysis

Prior to conducting the study, we performed a priori power analysis using statistical software (G*Power V3.1.9.7) to determine the required number of cadavers [30]. We determined a sample size of four stifle joints based on the following parameters: $\alpha = 0.05$, power = 0.8, and estimated effect size (d) = 2.5766667, derived from the mean and standard deviation (SD) observed in a pilot study involving four cadavers. However, the final sample included sixteen stifle joints from the pilot study, equally distributed among the two groups. Data were analyzed using SPSS software version 29 (IBM SPSS, Chicago, IL, USA). Additionally, the Kolmogorov–Smirnov test was employed to assess the normal distribution of continuous variables. Differences in data, excluding the number of intra-articular screws, were assessed using an independent t-test for each group. The number of intra-articular screws within each group was compared using the Mann–Whitney U test. A p-value of <0.05 was considered statistically significant.

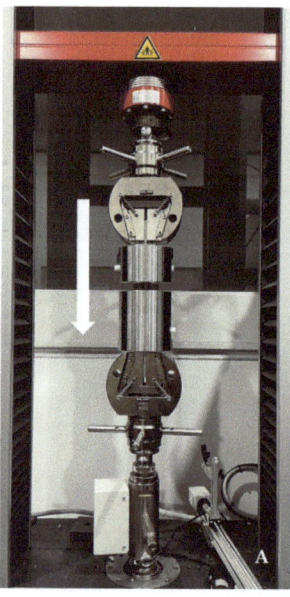
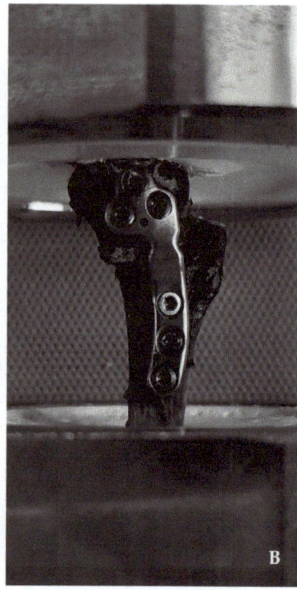

Figure 4. Photograph of the compression test. Mechanical testing stainless-steel jig affixed to the servo-hydraulic testing machine. A 3D resin jig is firmly positioned within a stainless-steel jig, and a compressive load is applied vertically downward (**A**). The tibia with the TPLO plate is securely fastened to the proximal and distal 3D resin jigs, ensuring that neither the plate nor the screws are embedded in plaster (**B**).

3. Results

3.1. Specimens

Sixteen hindlimbs were obtained from eight small-breed canine cadavers collected between March 2023 and September 2023. All cadavers weighed between 3 and 5 kg, including Chihuahua (3), Maltese (3), and mixed breeds (2). During the compression test, two hindlimbs had to be excluded from both the PCM–TPLO plate and the TPLO plate groups due to unintentional intraarticular screw placement.

3.2. Radiographic Measurements

The mean TPA and mMPTA values were measured from eight hindlimbs in each group (Table 1). In both groups, the postoperative TPA appeared to be 5°, as targeted, and no significant differences were found between the two groups ($p = 0.878$). There was also no significant difference in postoperative mMPTA between the two groups, and the changes before and after surgery were considered not statistically significant. However, in the PCM–TPLO plate group, there was a tendency for a decrease in postoperative mMPTA compared with preoperative mMPTA.

The number of screws within the joint was measured. Within the PCM–TPLO plate group, two dogs had one or two screws, respectively, entering the joint capsule (median, 1.5; range: 0–2). In contrast, the TPLO plate group showed no screws entering the joint capsule in any dog, and the difference between the two groups was not significant ($p = 0.442$).

The mean values of the bone–plate gap for each group are presented in Table 1. In the TPLO plate group, there was virtually no distance between the bone and plate, while the PCM–TPLO plate group exhibited a 1.9 mm gap, indicating a significant difference between the two groups.

The medialization distance and tibial osteotomy width were exclusively calculated for the PCM–TPLO plate group, demonstrating mean values and standard deviations of

2.275 ± 0.578 mm and 7.674 ± 0.763 mm, respectively. The calculated mean and standard deviation of the degree of medial translation were 0.30 and 0.08.

Compression tests for load to failure were conducted (Table 1). The plates of both groups were able to withstand forces > 700 N. Notably, no significant differences were observed between the two groups.

Table 1. Descriptive data for the TPLO and PCM–TPLO plate groups (mean ± SD).

Parameters	TPLO Plate Group		PCM–TPLO Plate Group		p Value
	Mean	SD	Mean	SD	
Preoperative TPA (°)	25.00	2.00	25.25	2.86	0.798
Postoperative TPA (°)	5.48	1.66	5.38	2.15	0.878
Preoperative mMPTA (°)	96.96	4.33	96.13	6.17	0.721
Postoperative mMPTA (°)	97.04	1.84	94.34	4.38	0.131
Bone–plate gap (mm)	0.59	0.54	1.90	0.44	0.001
Load to failure (N)	798.80	375.02	721.50	292.02	0.818

TPLO: tibial plateau leveling osteotomy, PCM–TPLO: pre-contoured tibial plateau leveling osteotomy, TPA: tibial plateau angle, mMPTA: mechanical medial proximal tibial angle.

4. Discussion

In our investigation, we conducted a comparative anatomical and biomechanical analysis using cadaver specimens to examine alignment and compression resistance between the traditional TPLO and PCM–TPLO plates. We evaluated the role of PCM–TPLO plates in mediating surgical outcomes. We found that pre-contouring the plate did not alter postoperative TPA or mMPTA, nor did it increase the incidence of screw penetration into the joint capsule. Although applying the PCM–TPLO plate led to a slightly larger bone–plate gap, this did not compromise the integrity of the plate strength.

TPLO surgery aims to counteract the forward-directed force on the tibia by adjusting the TPA [14,19]. Following surgery, a TPA of 5–6.5° should be maintained to prevent the tibia from moving forward while avoiding backward movement [17,25,31]. Clinically, gait improvement has been reported when the postoperative TPA is within 0–14° [32]. In our study, both the traditional TPLO and PCM–TPLO groups showed mean postoperative TPA values within these recommended parameters, with no marked difference between the two groups. These findings imply that plate contouring does not significantly affect the alignment of the tibial plateau. Therefore, the PCM–TPLO plate is likely to be effective in restoring normal leg function by protecting against both forward and backward thrust of the tibia.

Following TPLO and MPL corrective surgeries, instances of improper bone alignment have been reported, often attributed to suboptimal surgical techniques [24,31,33–35]. Misalignments, such as varus or valgus deformities, can be detected by measuring mMPTA [25,36]. According to previous studies, the standard value for mMPTA is around 95.1 ± 3.2° [33,36]. Consistent with this, our study found that both the control (TPLO) and PCM–TPLO plate groups maintained normal mMPTA values before and after surgery. However, a slight increase in postoperative mMPTA was observed in the PCM–TPLO group, contrary to the findings of previous research, but there was no statistical significance [14]. Although there was a minor adjustment, it stayed within the normal limits and showed no significant variance when compared with the standard TPLO plate group. From this, we infer that the PCM–TPLO plate can mediate the medial displacement of the proximal tibial segment while preserving the integrity of the limb's overall alignment.

The PCM–TPLO plate was designed to enable a medial shift of the tibia by 2 mm. A previous study noted that the application of a pre-contoured T-plate, designed for 2 mm medial displacement on a tibial model, typically resulted in a medial shift typically of 0.05–1 mm [20]. Our findings indicate a median medialization distance of 2.275 ± 0.58 mm, corresponding to approximately 30 ± 8% of the total length of the osteotomy site. The increased medialization observed could be attributed to the unique design of our plate and the effects of the surrounding soft tissue. Previous clinical successes in treatment of MPL grades I, II, and III were reported with an average medialization of 20% [14,20]. Furthermore, for optimal bone healing, the repositioned bone segment should cover at least 50% of the osteotomy gap [8]. Our data, demonstrating approximately 70% coverage, suggest that the PCM–TPLO plate facilitates suitable medialization without compromising bone healing. Nonetheless, further clinical studies are essential to fully ascertain the practical implications of these findings.

In our study, we observed a slightly larger gap between the bone and plate in the PCM–TPLO plate group compared with the standard TPLO plate group. Prior research suggested that a larger gap could decrease stability, raising concerns about the surgery's success [20]. However, our results revealed that the maximum force the plates could withstand did not significantly differ between groups. Both were capable of supporting average forces greater than 700 N, thereby highlighting the superior mechanical properties of the PCM–TPLO plate compared to those observed in previous studies [28,37]. This discrepancy may be attributable to the differences in plate designs used and methods for measuring force in our study. Considering the typical weight support of a dog's pelvic limb, which is approximately 20% of its body weight during the convalescent period after surgery, and the maximum force it experiences during activities such as trotting, the PCM–TPLO plate is estimated to handle approximately 70–80% of the dog's weight [28,38]. The other research indicated that peak force can significantly increase during more vigorous activities [39]. Based on these considerations, for a dog weighing 5 kg, the leg might be subjected to a load of approximately 100 N. Yet, our findings indicate that the PCM–TPLO plate can withstand considerably higher loads than this estimate, even with a 2 mm gap between the bone and the plate. Thus, we conclude that the PCM–TPLO plate remains a reliable and effective option for dogs weighing less than 5 kg, without any increased risk of failure. The adaptation of the PCM–TPLO plate for medialization has raised concerns regarding a potentially higher risk of screw penetration into the joint space. Originally, TPLO plates were designed to prevent the entry of screws into the joint due to the potential for intraarticular screws to inflict meniscal injuries or degenerative changes [40,41]. In the PCM–TPLO group, two screws were observed to penetrate the joint capsule. However, since the PCM–TPLO plate was designed similarly to conventional TPLO plates to prevent screws from intruding into the joint space, such occurrences are likely attributed to the surgeon. Additionally, there was no statistically significant difference between the two groups. Therefore, despite these instances, the use of the PCM–TPLO plate remains a viable surgical option, capable of withstanding significant loads without causing additional damage to the patient.

This study had several limitations. First, a limited number of cadaveric specimens were used. While cadavers provide a closer approximation to the physiological environment, it is important to note that such specimens may differ from the bones of living specimens regarding bone quality. Bones of living animals are typically more robust, and additional anatomical structures contribute to their ability to withstand force, implying that they might endure even higher loads. Additionally, the cadavers used in this study did not have concurrent orthopedic diseases of the stifle joint; thus, the pathological arthrokinematics regarding MPL could not be evaluated. Second, the mechanical test was conducted in only one direction, failing to reflect the combinations of forces from various directions that may occur in real-life scenarios. Because repetitive forces similar to clinical conditions were not assessed, further studies are required to evaluate the practical clinical applications of this technique. Finally, there are limitations to the procedure of lateralizing the tibial tuberosity. High-grade MPL with associated bone deformities, such as femoral varus deformity, decreased femoral anteversion angle, and tibial valgus deformity, cannot be adequately addressed solely by lateralization of the tibial tuberosity to realign the quadriceps muscles. These cases may necessitate additional corrective osteotomies.

5. Conclusions

We conducted a comparison between the conventional TPLO group and the PCM–TPLO plate group using cadavers of small dogs weighing between 3 and 5 kg. Our findings from postoperative radiography and mechanical tests confirmed that the PCM–TPLO plate effectively adjusts TPA without increasing the risk of additional complications. Furthermore, owing to its appropriate rearrangement effect of tibial tuberosity related to the extensor mechanism, this innovative plate is expected to emerge as a favorable surgical option for small-breed dogs with concurrent CCLR and MPL.

Author Contributions: Conceptualization, Y.R., E.J. and Y.J.; methodology E.J.; software, E.J.; validation, E.J. and Y.R.; formal analysis, E.J. and Y.J.; investigation, E.J.; resources, Y.J.; data curation, E.J.; writing—original draft preparation, E.J.; writing—review and editing, Y.R. and Y.J.; visualization, Y.R. and T.K.; supervision, Y.R.; project administration, D.L. and Y.R. Funding acquisition, Y.R. All authors have read and agreed to the published version of the manuscript.

Funding: This work was supported by the National Research Foundation of Korea (NRF) grant funded by the Korea government (MSIT) (RS-2023-00278989).

Institutional Review Board Statement: Ethical approval for the cadaver study protocol was not required by the Institutional Animal Care and Use Committee of Gyeongsang National University, as the cadavers were donated by their owners, and the euthanasia was unrelated to this study.

Informed Consent Statement: Not applicable.

Data Availability Statement: The original contributions presented in the study are included in the article, further inquiries can be directed to the corresponding author/s.

Conflicts of Interest: The authors declare no conflicts of interest.

References

1. LaFond, E.; Breur, G.J.; Austin, C.C. Breed susceptibility for developmental orthopedic diseases in dogs. *J. Am. Anim. Hosp. Assoc.* **2002**, *38*, 467–477. [CrossRef] [PubMed]
2. Ness, M.; Abercromby, R.; May, C.; Turner, B.; Carmichael, S. A survey of orthopaedic conditions in small animal veterinary practice in Britain. *Vet. Comp. Orthop. Traumatol.* **1996**, *9*, 43–52. [CrossRef]
3. Campbell, C.A.; Horstman, C.L.; Mason, D.R.; Evans, R.B. Severity of patellar luxation and frequency of concomitant cranial cruciate ligament rupture in dogs: 162 cases (2004–2007). *J. Am. Vet. Med. Assoc.* **2010**, *236*, 887–891. [CrossRef]
4. Gibbons, S.; Macias, C.; Tonzing, M.; Pinchbeck, G.; McKee, W. Patellar luxation in 70 large breed dogs. *J. Small Anim. Pract.* **2006**, *47*, 3–9. [CrossRef] [PubMed]
5. Hayes, A.G.; Boudrieau, R.J.; Hungerford, L.L. Frequency and distribution of medial and lateral patellar luxation in dogs: 124 cases (1982–1992). *J. Am. Vet. Med. Assoc.* **1994**, *205*, 716–720. [CrossRef] [PubMed]
6. Witsberger, T.H.; Villamil, J.A.; Schultz, L.G.; Hahn, A.W.; Cook, J.L. Prevalence of and risk factors for hip dysplasia and cranial cruciate ligament deficiency in dogs. *J. Am. Vet. Med. Assoc.* **2008**, *232*, 1818–1824. [CrossRef] [PubMed]
7. Arthurs, G.; Langley-Hobbs, S. Patellar luxation as a complication of surgical intervention for the management of cranial cruciate ligament rupture in dogs. *Vet. Comp. Orthop. Traumatol.* **2007**, *20*, 204–210. [CrossRef] [PubMed]
8. Kowaleski, M.P.; Boudrieau, R.J.; Pozzi, A. Stifle joint. In *Veterinary Surgery: Small Animal*, 2nd ed.; Tobias, K.M., Johnston, S.A., Eds.; Elsevier: St. Louis, MI, USA, 2012; Volume 1, pp. 1071–1168.
9. Panichi, E.; Cappellari, F.; Burkhan, E.; Principato, G.; Currenti, M.; Tabbì, M.; Macrì, F. Patient-Specific 3D-Printed Osteotomy Guides and Titanium Plates for Distal Femoral Deformities in Dogs with Lateral Patellar Luxation. *Animals* **2024**, *14*, 951. [CrossRef] [PubMed]
10. L'Eplattenier, H.; Montavon, P. Patellar luxation in dogs and cats: Pathogenesis and diagnosis. *Compendium* **2002**, *24*, 234–240.
11. Vasseur, P.B. Stifle Joint. In *Textbook of Small Animal Surgery*, 3rd ed.; Slatter, D.H., Ed.; Elsevier Health Sciences: Amsterdam, The Netherlands, 2003; Volume 1, pp. 2090–2132.
12. Langenbach, A.; Marcellin-Little, D.J. Management of concurrent patellar luxation and cranial cruciate ligament rupture using modified tibial plateau levelling. *J. Small Anim. Pract.* **2010**, *51*, 97–103. [CrossRef]
13. DeCamp, C.E.; Johnston, S.A.; Déjardin, L.M.; Schaefer, S.L. *Brinker, Piermattei and Flo's Handbook of Small Animal Orthopedics and Fracture Repair*, 5th ed.; Elsevier: St. Louis, MI, USA, 2015.

14. Flesher, K.; Beale, B.S.; Hudson, C.C. Technique and outcome of a modified tibial plateau levelling osteotomy for treatment of concurrent medial patellar luxation and cranial cruciate ligament rupture in 76 stifles. *Vet. Comp. Orthop. Traumatol.* **2019**, *32*, 026–032. [CrossRef]
15. Leonard, K.C.; Kowaleski, M.P.; Saunders, W.B.; McCarthy, R.J.; Boudrieau, R.J. Combined tibial plateau levelling osteotomy and tibial tuberosity transposition for treatment of cranial cruciate ligament insufficiency with concomitant medial patellar luxation. *Vet. Comp. Orthop. Traumatol.* **2016**, *29*, 536–540. [CrossRef] [PubMed]
16. Lampart, M.; Knell, S.; Pozzi, A. A new approach to treatment selection in dogs with cruciate ligament rupture: Patient-specific treatment recommendations. *Schweiz. Arch. Tierheilkd.* **2020**, *162*, 345–363. [CrossRef] [PubMed]
17. Slocum, B.; Slocum, T.D. Tibial plateau leveling osteotomy for repair of cranial cruciate ligament rupture in the canine. *Vet. Clin. North. Am. Small Anim. Pract.* **1993**, *23*, 777–795. [CrossRef] [PubMed]
18. Arthurs, G.I.; LANGLEY-HOBBS, S.J. Complications associated with corrective surgery for patellar luxation in 109 dogs. *Vet. Surg.* **2006**, *35*, 559–566. [CrossRef] [PubMed]
19. Birks, R.R.; Kowaleski, M.P. Combined tibial plateau levelling osteotomy and tibial tuberosity transposition: An ex vivo mechanical study. *Vet. Comp. Orthop. Traumatol.* **2018**, *31*, 124–130. [CrossRef] [PubMed]
20. Dallago, M.; Baroncelli, A.B.; Hudson, C.; Peirone, B.; De Bakker, E.; Piras, L.A. Effect of Plate Type on Tibial Plateau Levelling and Medialization Osteotomy for Treatment of Cranial Cruciate Ligament Rupture and Concomitant Medial Patellar Luxation in Small Breed Dogs: An In Vitro Study. *Vet. Comp. Orthop. Traumatol.* **2023**, *36*, 212–217. [CrossRef] [PubMed]
21. Kettleman, W.S. Ex Vivo Biomechanical Evaluation of a Novel Screw for Tibial Plateau Leveling Osteotomy. Master's Thesis, Mississippi State University, Starkville, MS, USA, 2022.
22. Curuci, E.H.; Bernardes, F.J.; Minto, B.W. Modified tibial plateau levelling osteotomy to treat lateral patellar luxation and cranial cruciate ligament deficiency in a dog. *Clin. Case Rep.* **2021**, *9*, e04365. [CrossRef] [PubMed]
23. Livet, V.; Taroni, M.; Ferrand, F.-X.; Carozzo, C.; Viguier, E.; Cachon, T. Modified triple tibial osteotomy for combined cranial cruciate ligament rupture, tibial deformities, or patellar luxation. *J. Am. Anim. Hosp. Assoc.* **2019**, *55*, 291–300. [CrossRef]
24. Windolf, M.; Leitner, M.; Schwieger, K.; Pearce, S.G.; Zeiter, S.; Schneider, E.; Johnson, K.A. Accuracy of fragment positioning after TPLO and effect on biomechanical stability. *Vet. Surg.* **2008**, *37*, 366–373. [CrossRef]
25. Slocum, B.; Devine, T. Cranial tibial thrust: A primary force in the canine stifle. *J. Am. Vet. Med. Assoc.* **1983**, *183*, 456–459. [PubMed]
26. Dismukes, D.I.; Tomlinson, J.L.; Fox, D.B.; Cook, J.L.; Song, K.J.E. Radiographic measurement of the proximal and distal mechanical joint angles in the canine tibia. *Vet. Surg.* **2007**, *36*, 699–704. [CrossRef] [PubMed]
27. Dismukes, D.I.; Tomlinson, J.L.; Fox, D.B.; Cook, J.L.; Witsberger, T.H. Radiographic measurement of canine tibial angles in the sagittal plane. *Vet. Surg.* **2008**, *37*, 300–305. [CrossRef] [PubMed]
28. Bordelon, J.; Coker, D.; Payton, M.; Rochat, M. An in vitro mechanical comparison of tibial plateau levelling osteotomy plates. *Vet. Comp. Orthop. Traumatol.* **2009**, *22*, 467–472. [CrossRef] [PubMed]
29. Sembenelli, G.; Souza, G.; Wittmaack, M.; Shimano, A.; Rocha, T.; Moraes, P.; Minto, B.; Dias, L. Biomechanical comparison of a modified TPLO plate, a locking compression plate, and plate-rod constructs applied medially in a proximal gap model in canine synthetic tibias. *Arq. Bras. Med. Vet. Zootec.* **2022**, *74*, 948–953. [CrossRef]
30. Faul, F.; Erdfelder, E.; Buchner, A.; Lang, A.-G. Statistical power analyses using G* Power 3.1: Tests for correlation and regression analyses. *Behav. Res. Methods* **2009**, *41*, 1149–1160. [CrossRef] [PubMed]
31. Warzee, C.C.; Dejardin, L.M.; Arnoczky, S.P.; Perry, R.L. Effect of tibial plateau leveling on cranial and caudal tibial thrusts in canine cranial cruciate–deficient stifles: An in vitro experimental study. *Vet. Surg.* **2001**, *30*, 278–286. [CrossRef] [PubMed]
32. Robinson, D.A.; Mason, D.R.; Evans, R.; Conzemius, M.G. The effect of tibial plateau angle on ground reaction forces 4–17 months after tibial plateau leveling osteotomy in Labrador Retrievers. *Vet. Surg.* **2006**, *35*, 294–299. [CrossRef] [PubMed]
33. Olimpo, M.; Piras, L.A.; Peirone, B. Pelvic limb alignment in small breed dogs: A comparison between affected and free subjects from medial patellar luxation. *Vet. Ital.* **2016**, *52*, 45–50. [CrossRef]
34. Reif, U.; Dejardin, L.M.; Probst, C.W.; DeCamp, C.E.; Flo, G.L.; Johnson, A.L. Influence of limb positioning and measurement method on the magnitude of the tibial plateau angle. *Vet. Surg.* **2004**, *33*, 368–375. [CrossRef]
35. Wheeler, J.L.; Cross, A.R.; Gingrich, W. In vitro effects of osteotomy angle and osteotomy reduction on tibial angulation and rotation during the tibial plateau-leveling osteotomy procedure. *Vet. Surg.* **2003**, *32*, 371–377. [CrossRef] [PubMed]
36. Aghapour, M.; Bockstahler, B.; Vidoni, B. Evaluation of the femoral and tibial alignments in dogs: A systematic review. *Animals* **2021**, *11*, 1804. [CrossRef]
37. Kloc, P.A.; Kowaleski, M.P.; Litsky, A.S.; Brown, N.O.; Johnson, K.A. Biomechanical comparison of two alternative tibial plateau leveling osteotomy plates with the original standard in an axially loaded gap model: An in vitro study. *Vet. Surg.* **2009**, *38*, 40–48. [CrossRef]
38. Duerr, F.M. *Canine Lameness*; John Wiley & Sons: Hoboken, NJ, USA, 2020.
39. Caporn, T.; Roe, S. Biomechanical evaluation of the suitability of monofilament nylon fishing and leader line for extra-articular stabilisation of the canine cruciate-deficient stifle. *Vet. Comp. Orthop. Traumatol.* **1996**, *9*, 126–133. [CrossRef]

40. Franklin, S.P.; Gilley, R.S.; Palmer, R.H. Meniscal injury in dogs with cranial cruciate ligament rupture. *Compend. Contin. Educ. Vet.* **2010**, *32*, E1–E10. [PubMed]
41. Polisetty, T.; DeVito, P.; Judd, H.; Malarkey, A.; Levy, J.C. Reverse shoulder arthroplasty for failed proximal humerus osteosynthesis with intramedullary allograft: A case series. *J. Shoulder Elb. Arthroplast.* **2020**, *4*, 2471549220925464. [CrossRef]

Disclaimer/Publisher's Note: The statements, opinions and data contained in all publications are solely those of the individual author(s) and contributor(s) and not of MDPI and/or the editor(s). MDPI and/or the editor(s) disclaim responsibility for any injury to people or property resulting from any ideas, methods, instructions or products referred to in the content.

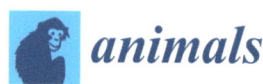

Case Report

Reconstruction of Bilateral Chronic Triceps Brachii Tendon Disruption Using a Suture-Mediated Anatomic Footprint Repair in a Dog

Jong-Pil Yoon [†], Hae-Beom Lee [†], Young-Jin Jeon, Dae-Hyun Kim, Seong-Mok Jeong and Jae-Min Jeong *

Department of Veterinary Surgery, College of Veterinary Medicine, Chungnam National University, 99, Daehak-ro, Yuseong-gu, Daejeon 34134, Republic of Korea; yjp0101@naver.com (J.-P.Y.); seatiger76@cnu.ac.kr (H.-B.L.); orangee0115@gmail.com (Y.-J.J.); vet1982@cnu.ac.kr (D.-H.K.); jsmok@cnu.ac.kr (S.-M.J.)
* Correspondence: klmie800@cnu.ac.kr; Tel.: +82-42-821-7404
† These authors contributed equally to this work.

Simple Summary: Chronic triceps brachii tendon disruptions in dogs can lead to significant lameness and discomfort, often requiring surgical intervention for effective treatment. This case report details the surgical reconstruction of bilateral chronic triceps brachii tendon disruptions in a 2-year-old female Pomeranian using a novel suture-mediated anatomic footprint repair technique. The technique, adapted from human medicine, involves creating a precise attachment of the tendon to the olecranon through specialized suturing and bone tunneling, which aims to restore normal anatomy and function. Following the surgery, the dog experienced significant improvement in forelimb function and was able to maintain a normal gait over a three-year follow-up period. This report demonstrates the successful application of a human surgical technique in veterinary medicine, providing a promising option for managing this rare but challenging condition in dogs. The technique's success suggests its potential utility in similar cases, offering insights that could benefit surgical practices in veterinary orthopedics.

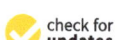

Citation: Yoon, J.-P.; Lee, H.-B.; Jeon, Y.-J.; Kim, D.-H.; Jeong, S.-M.; Jeong, J.-M. Reconstruction of Bilateral Chronic Triceps Brachii Tendon Disruption Using a Suture-Mediated Anatomic Footprint Repair in a Dog. *Animals* **2024**, *14*, 1687. https://doi.org/10.3390/ani14111687

Academic Editors: L. Miguel Carreira and João Alves

Received: 3 May 2024
Revised: 30 May 2024
Accepted: 4 June 2024
Published: 5 June 2024

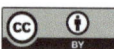

Copyright: © 2024 by the authors. Licensee MDPI, Basel, Switzerland. This article is an open access article distributed under the terms and conditions of the Creative Commons Attribution (CC BY) license (https://creativecommons.org/licenses/by/4.0/).

Abstract: A 2-year-old, intact female Pomeranian presented with bilateral forelimb lameness, characterized by the olecranon making contact with the ground. The patient experienced two separate incidents of falling, occurring four and three weeks before admission, respectively. Following each episode, non-weight-bearing lameness was initially observed in the left forelimb, followed by the development of crouch gait. Based on the physical examination, radiographic, and ultrasonographic findings, bilateral triceps brachii tendon disruption was diagnosed. Intraoperatively, excessive granulation tissue at the distal end of the tendon was excised. The footprint region of each triceps brachii tendon was decorticated with a high-speed burr until bleeding was observed. The triceps brachii tendon was reattached to completely cover its footprint on the olecranon using the Krackow suture technique. This method involves anchoring the suture through bone tunnels in the ulna. Trans-articular external skeletal fixation was applied to both forelimbs to immobile and stabilize the elbow joints for nine weeks. Subsequently, the dog gradually increased its walking activities while on a leash over a six-week period. At the three-year follow-up, the patient exhibited improved forelimb function and maintained a normal gait without signs of lameness. Suture-mediated anatomic footprint repair proved useful in this single case and may be an effective surgical alternative for the management of chronic triceps brachii tendon disruption in dogs.

Keywords: chronic triceps brachii tendon disruption; footprint repair; suture-mediated anatomic repair; Krackow suture; trans-articular external skeletal fixation; dog

1. Introduction

Disruption of the triceps brachii tendon, characterized by the tearing or detachment from its insertion on the olecranon, is rarely reported in small animals [1–5]. The etiology of this condition in small animals typically involves trauma, surgical interventions near the tendon attachment, and local or systemic corticosteroid injections, with trauma being the predominant cause [1,2]. Clinically, this condition is often manifested by non-weight-bearing lameness, soft tissue swelling, and pain upon palpation [1,2,4].

Diagnosis of triceps brachii tendon disruption relies on comprehensive physical and imaging examinations [1,2,6]. Physical examination may reveal a nodular formation and a palpable gap proximal to the olecranon of the affected limb. It is noteworthy that the squeeze test, which assesses tendon injury, may often be inconclusive [7]. Radiographic evaluations typically identify a flake sign at the triceps brachii tendon attachment, indicative of a potential avulsion injury [1,4]. Ultrasonography generally shows discontinuity or an abnormal appearance of the tendon fibers [5]. Magnetic resonance imaging (MRI) is considered the preferred method for diagnosing and differentiating complete from partial triceps brachii tendon disruption [7,8].

Given that tendon disruptions rarely heal with conservative therapy, surgical intervention is the standard treatment [2,9]. These disruptions can be categorized into three patterns as follows: myotendinous junction, central part of the tendon, and osseotendinous junction [1]. Disruption at the central part requires a tendon–tendon suture, while osseo-tendinous disruption necessitates a tendon–bone suture through bone tunnels [1,10]. Techniques for tendon–bone sutures include trans-osseous, suture anchor, and hybrid trans-osseous–suture anchor approaches [9,11]. The restoration of the anatomical footprint and the prevention of postoperative gap formation are crucial for tendon healing, as they significantly impact the biomechanical strength and speed of recovery [11–13]. In human medicine, traditional cruciate repair techniques utilized for tendon restoration have demonstrated a 21% recurrence rate because of the limited contact area between the tendon and bone. This limited contact reduces mechanical strength and delays healing. Consequently, techniques employing suture anchors are preferred for their strong holding strength and ease in reconstructing the footprint, which leads to successful outcomes [9,11].

Such footprint restoration techniques, while established in human medicine, have not been commonly applied in veterinary medicine, especially for small-breed dogs.

The application of anchors in small dogs can be challenging because of the limited bone availability at the olecranon [9]. Moreover, in chronic cases, excessive scar tissue, tendon retraction, and muscle atrophy can occur following tendon degeneration, resulting in a large gap [3,14–17]. The poor tissue quality of tendon ends may also adversely affect the suture's holding strength [3]. Therefore, a trans-osseous technique that can mechanically withstand long-term stress and prevent gap formation while reconstructing the footprint seems indicated for dogs with chronic triceps brachii tendon disruption. This report describes the successful outcome of surgical treatment using a novel suture-mediated anatomic footprint repair in a dog with chronic bilateral triceps brachii tendon disruptions.

2. Case Description

A 2-year-old, 4.5 kg, intact female Pomeranian was referred to a veterinary medicine teaching hospital with bilateral open wounds (Video S1, Figure 1A) at the olecranon region. The dog presented with a history of bilateral forelimb lameness and crouch gait (Figure 1B) as follows: four weeks in the left forelimb and three weeks in the right forelimb, each following a fall from a height. Physical examination revealed a pain response and nodular formation in the proximal region of the olecranon, with no extension response during the triceps brachii squeeze test. Radiographs revealed radiolucent opacities on both sides of the olecranon (Figure 2A,B), and ultrasonography identified defects (Figure 3A,B) at the triceps brachii tendon and olecranon junction, accompanied by inflammation and edema. Notably, the distal end of the proximal tendon appeared hyperechoic compared with the normal tendon. Based on the diagnosis of bilateral triceps brachii tendon disruption, believed to be of traumatic origin, and with the exact cause remaining open to interpretation, surgical repair was indicated. The initial management of the open wounds involved sugar dressing and debridement. Pre-anesthetic evaluation through blood samples, assessing electrolytes, and complete blood count (CBC), revealed all values within normal limits.

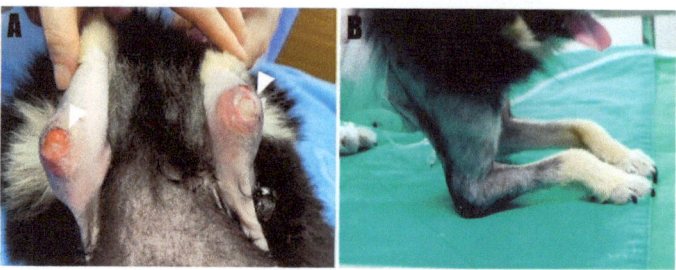

Figure 1. (**A**) Chronic ulceration wounds were evident on the bilateral elbow (arrowhead). (**B**) The dog exhibited a crouching posture, indicative of an abnormal standing.

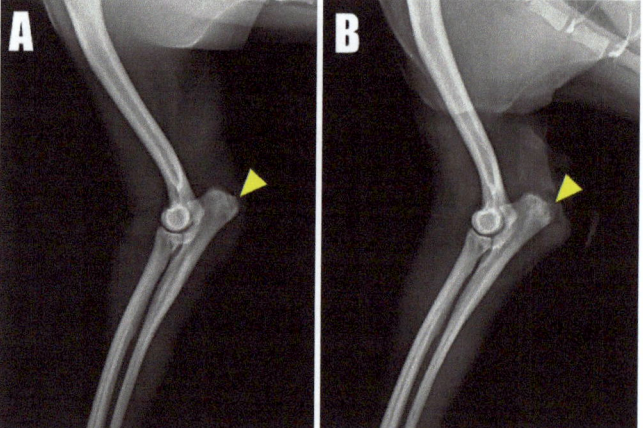

Figure 2. Radiolucent opacity (yellow arrowhead) was visible on the olecranon in radiographic images of the (**A**) right and (**B**) left forelimbs.

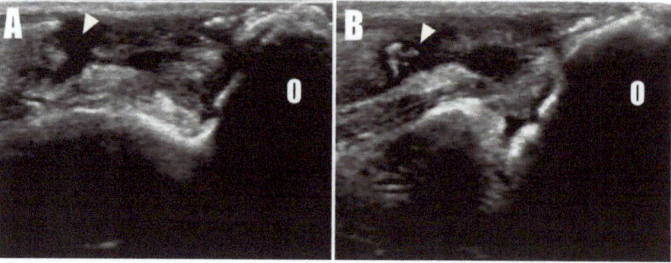

Figure 3. Disruption of the triceps brachii tendon (arrowhead) from the olecranon (O) was confirmed in ultrasonographic images of the (**A**) right and (**B**) left sides.

The surgical procedures were performed with informed consent from the owner. The dog was premedicated with midazolam (0.2 mg/kg, IV) and ketamine (0.5 mg/kg, IV), followed by induction with propofol (6 mg/kg, IV) and maintenance of general anesthesia with isoflurane and oxygen via a rebreathing circuit. Analgesia was provided by constant rate infusion of remifentanil (0.1–0.3 ug/kg), and cefazolin (22 mg/kg, IV) was administered for prophylaxis 30 min before incision and repeated every 90 min for a total of three doses.

The dog was placed in dorsal recumbency with bilateral elbow joints placed uppermost. To approach the humeroulnar part, a caudolateral approach to the olecranon was made [2]. Fascia were incised and retracted, exposing the triceps brachii tendon and olecranon. Granulation tissue was meticulously debrided with a rongeur and scalpel blade, and the triceps brachii footprint (Figure 3A) on the olecranon was decorticated using an electrically powered oval-shaped burr (Core, Stryker, Kalamazoo, MI, USA) to promote tendon-to-bone healing [12]. The bone tunnel preparation and suture repair technique were adopted from previously reported all-suture repair methods in human medicine, with slight modification. Initially, the origins of the anconeus and flexor carpi ulnaris were elevated from the olecranon to facilitate proper bone tunneling (Figure 4A). Subsequently, two tunnels were created on the craniomedial and craniolateral aspects of the footprint. These tunnels were drilled at 40° relative to the proximal anatomic axis of the olecranon, directed caudodistally, using an aiming device and a 1.2 mm Kirschner wire (K-wire) (Figures 4B and 5A,B). The tunnels were drilled to intersect in a "cross" pattern. Similarly, two additional tunnels were created cranially compared to the initial pair, angled approximately 60 degrees to the proximal anatomical axis of the olecranon, to maintain the cross pattern (Figures 4B and 5C,D). The final bone tunnel was drilled transversely across the long axis of the ulna using a 1.6 mm K-wire, serving as an anchorage point for the suture knots (Figures 4C and 5E).

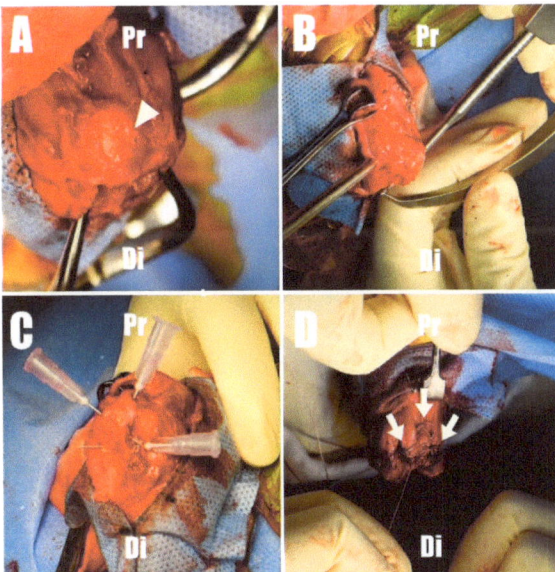

Figure 4. (**A**) The footprint (arrowhead) of the olecranon was decorticated to promote tendon-to-bone healing. (**B**) A C-guide was employed to create a caudal suture hole at the footprint. (**C**) The subsequent process involved the careful marking of the suture hole positions for verification using 26G needles. (**D**) The final stage involved the application of three Krackow stitches (arrow) for tendon repair with 2-0 FiberWire. Pr, proximal; Di, distal.

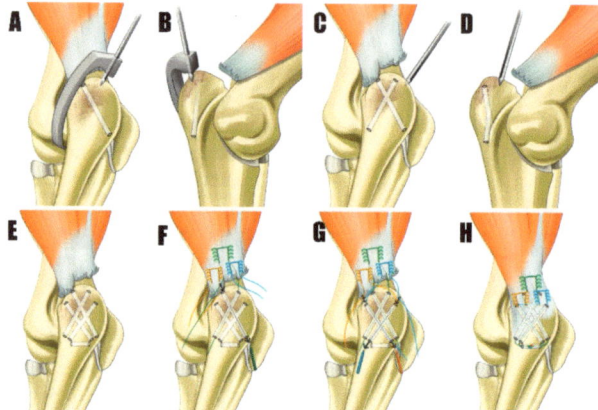

Figure 5. (**A,B**) These tunnels were originated cranially, employing a C-guide to maintain the integrity of the cross pattern. (**C,D**) Kirschner wire was used to meticulously create bone tunnels in a cross pattern within the footprint region, directed in craniomedial and craniolateral orientations for suture placement. (**E**) The final bone tunnel was created transversely along the ulna's long axis. (**F**) The application of three Krakow sutures to the tendon, with the most proximal suture (green) passed through the cranial bone tunnel using a suture passer, exiting laterally and medially to enable crossing. (**G**) Two distal sutures (brown and blue) were passed through the caudal bone tunnels. Each suture's inner strand was threaded through the bone tunnel on the opposite side to create a crossing configuration. (**H**) All sutures were passed and crossed through the transverse bone tunnel, forming a knot.

A 2-0 size FiberWire suture (Arthrex, Naples, FL, USA) was employed using a locking Krackow technique (Figure 4D), positioned at the proximal aspect of the tendon. This ensured that enough tendon distal to the suture exits was left to completely cover the triceps brachii footprint. The suture ends were passed through the most craniomedial and craniolateral bone tunnels in a crossing pattern, with the lateral suture end entering the craniolateral hole and exiting caudomedially, and the medial suture ends entering the craniomedial hole and exiting caudolaterally (Figure 5E). Second and third locking Krackow sutures were placed parallel on each medial and lateral side of the triceps brachii tendon's distal end (Figure 5F). The medial ends of each suture were passed through the caudally positioned craniomedial hole, and the lateral ends through the caudally positioned craniolateral hole, using a suture passer. Three limbs of the suture were threaded through the transverse tunnel (Figure 5H). The suture exiting the proximal aspect of the tendon was tied first, with the elbow in full extension to ensure anatomical reconstruction. After the initial tie, the sutures emerging distally were matched and tied accordingly.

Saline lavage was performed on the surgical site, which was then swabbed for culture and sensitivity tests before routine closure. Following closure, a trans-articular external skeletal fixator (TAESF) was applied for joint immobilization. A circular ring was placed on the radius using two 1.0 mm K-wires. Two 2.4 mm Duraface ESF end thread pins (IMEX Veterinary InC., Longview, TX, USA) were inserted into the humerus and connected with lateral connecting bars. The elbow joint angle was immobilized at 150 degrees to reduce tension on the tenorrhaphy. The contralateral limb underwent identical treatment.

Postoperative radiographs and ultrasound images (Figure 6) were taken to confirm the position and connectivity (Figure 7) of the tendon on the olecranon. On the right side (Figure 6A), the transverse hole was observed to be close to the caudal cortex, while the remaining bone tunnels were confirmed to have been drilled as intended. For analgesia, remifentanil was continued for three days postoperatively at 0.1~0.3 ug/kg/min with constant rate infusion. The other postoperative therapy including antibiotics (amoxicillin and clavulanic acid, 12.5 mg/kg BID, for 14 days/Clindamycin, 11 mg/kg BID, for 14 days), NSAID (meloxicam, 0.1 mg/kg SID for 14 days), and gastrointestinal protectant (esomeprazole, 1 mg/kg SID for 14 days) were administered.

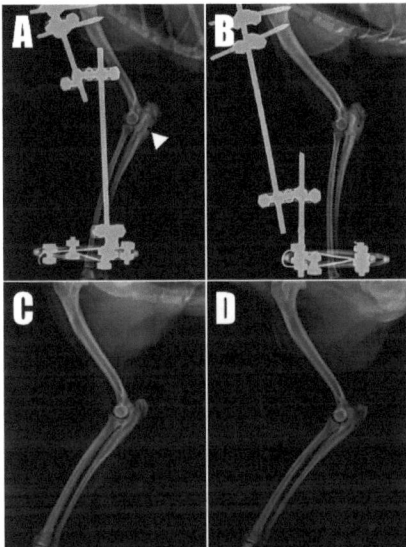

Figure 6. Immediate postoperative radiograph of the (**A**) right forelimb showing the transverse hole (arrowhead) in the caudal aspect of the ulna. (**B**) A corresponding image of the of the left forelimb. Six-month postoperative radiograph of the (**C**) right and (**D**) left forelimb.

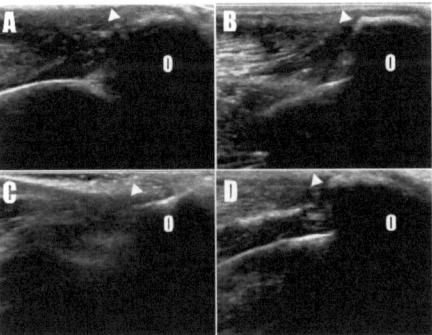

Figure 7. Ultrasound images taken two weeks postoperatively of the (**A**) right and (**B**) left forelimbs confirm the attachment of the triceps brachii tendon (arrowhead) to the olecranon (O). Similar findings were observed in the ultrasound images six months postoperatively on the (**C**) right and (**D**) left forelimbs.

Immediate postoperative weight-bearing was observed. The patient was discharged two weeks postoperatively with instructions for cage rest. To prevent joint ankylosis, the bolts and nuts were slightly loosened, and the trans-articular external skeletal fixator (TAESF) was progressively released six weeks postoperatively to allow a limited range of motion of about 10 degrees. The range of motion (ROM) was gradually increased to a maximum of 30 degrees, and ultimately, the TAESF was removed nine weeks postoperatively. The limbs were then supported in a Spica splint for an additional two weeks.

Radiography (Figure 6C,D) and ultrasonography (Figure 7C,D) six months postoperatively confirmed that the transverse hole of the right side healed without any complications, and the bilateral triceps brachii tendons were well-maintained and attached to the olecranon, with no specific changes in internal echogenicity or echotexture. MRI (Figure 8) showed mild inflammatory changes near the suture knot and fibrotic scar tissue within the tendon but confirmed firm attachment of the tendon to the olecranon. Three years following the surgery, the patient exhibited no signs of functional loss (Video S2) or pain, confirming the long-term success of the treatment. The owner expressed satisfaction with the clinical outcomes.

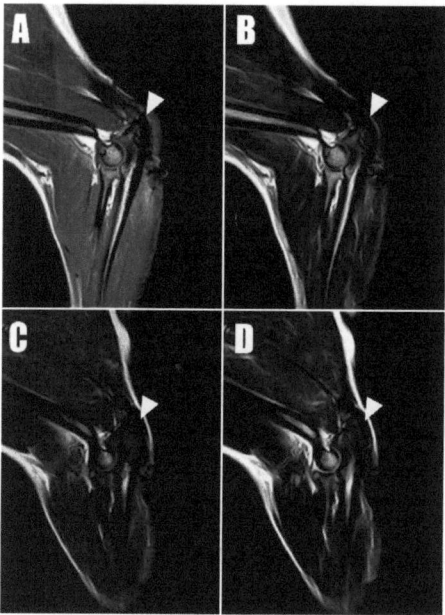

Figure 8. Postoperative magnetic resonance imaging (MRI) taken one year postoperatively captured (**A**) T1-weighted and (**B**) T2-weighted sagittal images of the right triceps brachii tendon, along with (**C**) T1- T1-weighted and (**D**) T2-weighted sagittal images of the left of triceps brachii tendon. These images demonstrate low signal intensity on both T1 and T2 sequences, indicating intact connectivity of the tendon.

3. Discussion

A suture-mediated footprint anatomic repair of the triceps brachii tendon was successfully utilized to restore full and recurrence-free forelimb function in a dog. The significance of this case lies in its novel application of a suture technique, previously documented in the human medical literature but adapted here for veterinary use with modification. The procedure resulted in excellent limb function as evidenced by long-term follow-up. This positive outcome, although in only a single case, is encouraging, and the technique can be recommended in similar cases.

Triceps brachii tendon disruption, though rare in small animals, poses significant challenges because of its varied etiology and the complexity of surgical repairs [1–5]. In humans, triceps brachii tendon injuries are attributed to multiple factors, including trauma, anabolic steroid use, weightlifting [18], local steroid injections [19], and a range of systemic conditions. Similarly, in veterinary medicine, tendon disruptions have been reported following local steroid injections [5], and breed-specific differences cannot be ruled out. Notably, triceps brachii tendon disruptions have been observed in Pomeranians [2,4], highlighting the need for further research to understand potential breed-specific predispositions. In our Pomeranian case, the bilateral nature of the tendon disruption, precipitated by falls, does not entirely exclude the possibility that degenerative changes, similar to those seen in cranial cruciate ligament disease, were exacerbated by minor trauma [20]. Additionally, inadequate vascularization [21] or a smaller insertion site at the tendon's insertion compared with other regions could also be contributing factors to this disruption. Further research is needed to explore these aspects comprehensively.

In human medicine, triceps brachii tendon disruptions typically occur at the osseotendinous junction, where several repair strategies are employed, including trans-osseous, suture anchor, and hybrid approaches [10,22]. However, traditional trans-osseous repairs, which have a notable failure rate of approximately 21%, often fail to adequately cover the triceps brachii footprint, leading to higher failure rates compared with those using suture anchors [9,11]. These anchors, however, present limitations in small dogs because of the risk of bone fracture [9]. Importantly, anatomic footprint repairs have demonstrated the highest average failure yield load, emphasizing their effectiveness. Specifically, when comparing gap formation rates, which are crucial for the tendon's healing process, traditional methods exhibit a high rate of 69%, suture anchors have a rate of 52%, and anatomic footprint repairs show a significantly lower rate of 14% [13,17]. In light of these factors, the consideration of anatomic footprint repair and meticulous surgical preparation is essential when addressing tendon disruptions at the osseo-tendinous junction [9]. In this case, a suture-mediated anatomic footprint repair technique, developed for human medicine, was adapted for a chronic condition in a dog, utilizing triple Krackow stitches and modifying the attachment method with two additional holes. This modification expanded the attachment surface area, enhancing durability and reducing gap formation.

The decision to use a trans-articular external skeletal fixator (TAESF) over external coaptation was influenced by the dog's history of pressure sores and the need for surgical wound access. TAESF, typically applied for three to eight weeks, in this case, was maintained for approximately nine weeks because of the chronic bilateral rupture, which anticipated a slow healing process. Adjustments were made six weeks postoperatively to prevent elbow joint ankylosis by allowing limited movement.

Tendon structural integrity and musculotendinous change are best evaluated by magnetic resonance imaging (MRI). In the late stages of tendon healing, tendons typically exhibit low signal intensity across T1- and T2-weighted MRI sequences [23]. In the current case, the bilateral triceps brachii tendons at their attachment to the olecranon demonstrated low signal intensity in all sequences at the one-year postoperative evaluation, with the exception of mild inflammatory changes observed near the suture knots and surrounding scar tissues.

This case report, while offering some insights, is constrained by several limitations. Firstly, it is based on a singular case, which may limit the broader applicability of our findings. Without the support of more extensive diagnostic procedures, such as a biopsy, we acknowledge our limitations in conclusively identifying other potential causes. Furthermore, there is a recognized need for more comprehensive biomechanical studies to compare the efficacy of traditional repair techniques, suture anchors, and the anatomic footprint repair technique applied in this case. Finally, the investigation into the triceps brachii tendon's footprint area in dogs remains an uncharted area of study, suggesting a valuable opportunity for future research to fill this gap in the veterinary literature.

4. Conclusions

In conclusion, this case report details the surgical management and postoperative care of a dog with chronic bilateral triceps brachii tendon disruption, illustrating the importance of suture-mediated anatomic footprint repair combined with trans-articular external skeletal fixation (TAESF). It underscores the critical role of understanding and preserving the tendon's footprint during reconstruction for successful recovery. However, it also acknowledges the gap in our current knowledge regarding the precise extent of the triceps brachii tendon's footprint area in dogs, emphasizing the need for further research in this area to enhance surgical outcomes in similar cases.

Supplementary Materials: The following supporting information can be downloaded at https://www.mdpi.com/article/10.3390/ani14111687/s1, Video S1: Preoperative crouch gait. The olecranon made contact with the ground while walking. To prevent further damage to an open wound, the lib was supported with a sling during the gait assessment. Video S2: Postoperative gait. A normal gait has been consistently maintained for three years postoperatively.

Author Contributions: Conceptualization, J.-P.Y., Y.-J.J., H.-B.L. and J.-M.J.; methodology, J.-P.Y., H.-B.L. and J.-M.J.; software, J.-P.Y., Y.-J.J and H.-B.L.; validation, J.-P.Y., Y.-J.J., D.-H.K., S.-M.J., H.-B.L. and J.-M.J.; formal analysis, J.-P.Y.; investigation, J.-P.Y. and H.-B.L.; resources, J.-P.Y., Y.-J.J., H.-B.L. and J.-M.J.; data curation, J.-P.Y., D.-H.K. and S.-M.J.; writing—original draft preparation, J.-P.Y., H.-B.L. and J.-M.J.; writing—review and editing, J.-P.Y., Y.-J.J., D.-H.K., S.-M.J., H.-B.L. and J.-M.J.; visualization, J.-P.Y.; supervision, H.-B.L. and J.-M.J.; projection administration, H.-B.L and J.-M.J. All authors have read and agreed to the published version of the manuscript.

Funding: This research received no external funding.

Institutional Review Board Statement: Ethical review and approval were not required because this study is a case report of an examination and surgery for the purpose of treating the patient, and no action contrary to treatment was performed.

Informed Consent Statement: Written informed consent was obtained from the owner of the animal involved in this study.

Data Availability Statement: The original contributions presented in this study are included in this article/the Supplementary Materials. Further inquiries can be directed to the corresponding author.

Acknowledgments: This work was supported by the research fund of Chungnam National University.

Conflicts of Interest: The authors declare no conflicts of interest. The funders had no role in the design of this study; in the collection, analyses, or interpretation of the data; in the writing of this manuscript; or in the decision to publish the results.

References

1. Earley, N.F.; Ellse, G.; Wallace, A.M.; Parsons, K.J.; Voss, K.; Pugliese, L.C.; Moores, A.P.; Whitelock, R.; Stork, C.; Langley-Hobbs, S.J.; et al. Complications and outcomes associated with 13 cases of triceps tendon disruption in dogs and cats (2003–2014). *Vet. Rec.* **2018**, *182*, 108. [CrossRef] [PubMed]
2. Echigo, R.; Fujita, A.; Nishimura, R.; Mochizuki, M. Triceps brachii tendon injury in four Pomeranians. *J. Vet. Med. Sci.* **2018**, *80*, 772–777. [CrossRef]
3. Wood, C.J.; Cashmore, R.G. Repair of a Chronic Triceps Tendon Rupture in a Dog Using an Autogenous Thoracolumbar Fascia Onlay Graft. *Vet. Comp. Orthop. Traumatol.* **2021**, *4*, e32–e36. [CrossRef]
4. Yoon, H.-Y.; Jeong, S.-W. Traumatic triceps tendon avulsion in a dog: Magnetic resonance imaging and surgical management evaluation. *J. Vet. Med. Sci.* **2013**, *75*, 1375–1377. [CrossRef] [PubMed]
5. Garcia-Fernandez, P.; Martín, P.Q.; Mayenco, A.; Gardoqui, M.; Calvo, I. Surgical management and follow-up of triceps tendon avulsion after repeated local infiltration of steroids: Two cases. *Vet. Comp. Orthop. Traumatol.* **2014**, *27*, 405–410. [CrossRef] [PubMed]
6. Liu, S.; Xie, Y.; Chen, Q.; Sun, Y.; Ding, Z.; Zhang, Y.; Chen, S.; Chen, J. Tendon healing progression evaluated with magnetic resonance imaging signal intensity and its correlation with clinical outcomes within 1 year after rotator cuff repair with the suture-bridge technique. *Am. J. Sports Med.* **2020**, *48*, 697–705. [CrossRef]
7. Tom, J.A.; Kumar, N.S.; Cerynik, D.L.; Mashru, R.; Parrella, M.S. Diagnosis and treatment of triceps tendon injuries: A review of the literature. *Clin. J. Sport. Med.* **2014**, *24*, 197–204. [CrossRef] [PubMed]
8. Bennett, M.P.; Silver, G.; Tromblee, T.; Kohler, R.; Frem, D.; Glass, E.N.; Kent, M. Case report: Nonsimultaneous bilateral triceps tendon rupture and surgical repair in a healthy dog. *Front. Vet. Sci.* **2024**, *10*, 1294395. [CrossRef]
9. Anderson, C.N. All-Suture Anatomic Footprint Repair of the Distal Triceps Tendon. *Arthrosc. Tech.* **2020**, *9*, e2013–e2019. [CrossRef]
10. Yeh, P.C.; El Attrache, N.S.; Mazzocca, A.; Katie, V.; Sethi, P.M. Distal Triceps Tendon Repair Using an Anatomic Footprint Repair. *Tech. Shoulder Elb. Surg.* **2011**, *12*, 62–66. [CrossRef]
11. Yeh, P.C.; Stephens, K.T.; Solovyova, O.; Obopilwe, E.; Smart, L.R.; Mazzocca, A.D.; Sethi, P.M. The Distal Triceps Tendon Footprint and a Biomechanical Analysis of 3 Repair Techniques. *Am. J. Sports Med.* **2010**, *38*, 1025–1033. [CrossRef] [PubMed]

12. Nakagawa, H.; Morihara, T.; Fujiwara, H.; Kabuto, Y.; Sukenari, T.; Kida, Y.; Furukawa, R.; Arai, Y.; Matsuda, K.-I.; Kawata, M.; et al. Effect of footprint preparation on tendon-to-bone healing: A histologic and biomechanical study in a rat rotator cuff repair model. *Arthroscopy* **2017**, *33*, 1482–1492. [CrossRef] [PubMed]
13. Wilson, L.; Banks, T.; Luckman, P.; Smith, B. Biomechanical evaluation of double K rackow sutures versus the three-loop pulley suture in a canine gastrocnemius tendon avulsion model. *Aust. Vet. J.* **2014**, *92*, 427–432. [CrossRef] [PubMed]
14. Us, A.K.; Bilgin, S.S.; Aydin, T.; Mergen, E. Repair of neglected Achilles tendon ruptures: Procedures and functional results. *Arch. Orthop. Trauma. Surg.* **1997**, *116*, 408–411. [CrossRef]
15. Ibrahim, S.A.R. Surgical treatment of chronic Achilles tendon rupture. *J. Foot Ankle Surg.* **2009**, *48*, 340–346. [CrossRef]
16. Buttin, P.; Goin, B.; Cachon, T.; Viguier, E. Repair of tendon disruption using a novel synthetic fiber implant in dogs and cats: The surgical procedure and three case reports. *Vet. Med. Int.* **2020**, *2020*, 4146790. [CrossRef] [PubMed]
17. Gelberman, R.H.; Boyer, M.I.; Brodt, M.D.; Winters, S.C.; Silva, M.J. The Effect of Gap Formation at the Repair Site on the Strength and Excursion of Intrasynovial Flexor Tendons. An Experimental Study on The Early Stages of Tendon-Healing in Dogs*. *J. Bone Jt. Surg. Am.* **1999**, *81*, 975–982. [CrossRef] [PubMed]
18. Sollender, J.L.; Rayan, G.M.; Barden, G.A. Triceps tendon rupture in weight lifters. *J. Shoulder Elbow Surg.* **1998**, *7*, 151–153. [CrossRef] [PubMed]
19. Stannard, J.P.; Bucknell, A.L. Rupture of the triceps tendon associated with steroid injections. *Am. J. Sports Med.* **1993**, *21*, 482–485. [CrossRef]
20. Ichinohe, T.; Kanno, N.; Harada, Y.; Yogo, T.; Tagawa, M.; Soeta, S.; Amasaki, H.; Hara, Y. Degenerative changes of the cranial cruciate ligament harvested from dogs with cranial cruciate ligament rupture. *J. Vet. Med. Sci.* **2015**, *77*, 761–770. [CrossRef]
21. Jopp, I.; Reese, S. Morphological and biomechanical studies on the common calcaneal tendon in dogs. *Vet. Comp. Orthop. Traumatol.* **2009**, *22*, 119–124. [CrossRef] [PubMed]
22. Van Riet, R.P.; Morrey, B.F.; Ho, E.; O'Driscoll, S.W. Surgical Treatment of Distal Triceps Ruptures. *J. Bone Jt. Surg. Am.* **2003**, *85*, 1961–1967. [CrossRef] [PubMed]
23. Joannas, G.; Arrondo, G.; Casola, L.; Drago, J.; Barousse, R.; Rossi, I.; Rammelt, S. Value of magnetic resonance imaging in monitoring Achilles tendon healing after percutaneous suture using the Dresden technique. *Fuß Sprunggelenk* **2019**, *17*, 210–218. [CrossRef]

Disclaimer/Publisher's Note: The statements, opinions and data contained in all publications are solely those of the individual author(s) and contributor(s) and not of MDPI and/or the editor(s). MDPI and/or the editor(s) disclaim responsibility for any injury to people or property resulting from any ideas, methods, instructions or products referred to in the content.

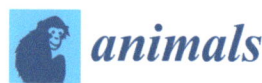

Case Report

Reconstruction of the Quadriceps Extensor Mechanism with a Calcaneal Tendon–Bone Allograft in a Dog with a Resorbed Tibial Tuberosity Fracture

Hyunho Kim [1,†], Haebeom Lee [1,†], Daniel D. Lewis [2], Jaemin Jeong [1], Gyumin Kim [3] and Youngjin Jeon [1,*]

[1] Department of Veterinary Surgery, College of Veterinary Medicine, Chungnam National University, Daejeon 34134, Republic of Korea; wwkhww@hanmail.net (H.K.); seatiger76@cnu.ac.kr (H.L.); klmie800@cnu.ac.kr (J.J.)
[2] Department of Small Animal Clinical Sciences, College of Veterinary Medicine, University of Florida, Gainesville, FL 32610, USA; lewisda@ufl.edu
[3] College of Veterinary Medicine, Jeonbuk National University, Iksan 54596, Republic of Korea; vetkgm@naver.com
* Correspondence: orangee0115@cnu.ac.kr
† These authors contributed equally to this work.

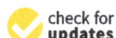

Citation: Kim, H.; Lee, H.; Lewis, D.D.; Jeong, J.; Kim, G.; Jeon, Y. Reconstruction of the Quadriceps Extensor Mechanism with a Calcaneal Tendon–Bone Allograft in a Dog with a Resorbed Tibial Tuberosity Fracture. *Animals* **2024**, *14*, 2315. https://doi.org/10.3390/ani14162315

Academic Editors: L. Miguel Carreira and João Alves

Received: 19 June 2024
Revised: 7 August 2024
Accepted: 8 August 2024
Published: 9 August 2024

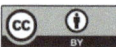

Copyright: © 2024 by the authors. Licensee MDPI, Basel, Switzerland. This article is an open access article distributed under the terms and conditions of the Creative Commons Attribution (CC BY) license (https://creativecommons.org/licenses/by/4.0/).

Simple Summary: This case report describes the surgical technique and clinical outcome of reconstructing the quadriceps mechanism using a composite frozen calcaneal tendon–bone block allograft in a dog which had resorption of the tibial tuberosity following complications resultant from a tibial tuberosity transposition procedure. In this case, a dog exhibited chronic lameness due to the resorption of the tibial tuberosity following surgical correction of a medial patella luxation. To address these issues, a novel surgical procedure was employed using a composite calcaneal tendon–bone block allograft. The graft reconstructed the tibial tuberosity and facilitated reattachment of the patellar tendon. The surgery promptly restored the quadriceps extensor mechanism, enabling the dog to bear weight on the affected limb within 2 weeks. Twenty-nine months later, the dog had satisfactory limb function without recurrence of patella luxation. This case demonstrates the effectiveness of using a calcaneal tendon–bone allograft to restore the quadriceps extensor mechanism in dogs with irreparable tibial tuberosity fracture.

Abstract: A non-reducible tibial tuberosity fracture is a rare complication of tibial tuberosity transposition performed during correcting of medial patella luxation (MPL) in dogs. This condition severely disrupts the quadriceps extensor mechanism, leading to significant pelvic limb lameness. An 11-year-old, 1.8 kg spayed female Yorkshire Terrier sustained a comminuted left tibial tuberosity fracture during surgical correction of an MPL. Six months after surgery, the dog was markedly lame and unable to extend the left stifle. Radiographs revealed patella alta and resorption of the fragmented tibial tuberosity. A composite frozen allogeneic calcaneal tendon–bone block was utilized to reconstruct the tibial tuberosity and reattach the patellar ligament. Initial postoperative radiographs confirmed restoration of a normal patellar ligament to patella length ratio (1.42). Both the allogeneic bone used for tibial tuberosity reconstruction and the tendon used to reattach the patellar ligament were successfully integrated. The dog regained satisfactory limb function without recurrence of patella luxation, as reported by the owners 29 months postoperatively. The use of a calcaneal tendon–bone allograft effectively restored the functional integrity of the quadriceps extensor mechanism, providing a viable option for addressing quadriceps insufficiency resulting from the loss of the osseous tibial insertion.

Keywords: tibia tuberosity reconstruction; tendon injury; allogenic tendon transplantation; quadriceps mechanism restoration

1. Introduction

Unrepairable tibial tuberosity fractures are a rare but significant complication following tibial tuberosity transposition performed to address medial patella luxation (MPL) in affected dogs [1,2]. Fractures of the tuberosity can occur if the tuberosity segment is too small: either while performing the osteotomy or during the placement of Kirschner wires intended to stabilize the transposed tuberosity [1,2]. Fragmentation of the tibial tuberosity can severely impair the quadriceps extensor mechanism and limb function. Restoration of quadriceps function can be challenging as the remaining bone fragments attached to the patellar ligament may be too small to accommodate adequate fixation. Consequently, non-reducible tibial tuberosity fractures may necessitate a salvage procedure, such as stifle arthrodesis or amputation [3].

The calcaneal tendon has high tensile strength and a long, broad aponeuroses, making calcaneal tendon allografts a suitable structural and functional replacement option for ligament reconstruction in human patients [4–6]. The allogenic tendon acts as a scaffold to facilitate cellular migration and functional ingrowth, which eventually leads to parenchymal remodeling and integration with the native tissues, yielding functionality [4,6]. An attached segment of calcaneal bone is often harvested with the tendon to enable osseous fixation of the graft [7,8]. These attributes have contributed to the effective use of calcaneal tendon–bone allografts in human patients for various ligament reconstructions, including addressing anterior cruciate ligament, calcaneal tendon, medial collateral ligament, and biceps tendon insufficiencies [9–11]. Several studies have described the effective use of calcaneal tendon–bone allografts to manage quadriceps extensor mechanism insufficiency in human patients with patellar tendon rupture [12–14]. While there are a couple of reports detailing the use of calcaneal tendon allografts to augment tendon-to-tendon repairs in dogs with patellar tendon injuries [15,16], the application of a calcaneal tendon–bone allograft to address irreparable tibial tuberosity fractures has not been reported.

This case report describes the surgical technique and clinical outcome associated with the use of a composite calcaneal tendon–bone block allograft to restore the quadriceps extensor mechanism in a dog with chronic lameness ascribed to an unrepairable tibial tuberosity fracture. Implantation of a calcaneal tendon–bone block allograft may be a reasonable option to address non-reducible tibial tuberosity fractures.

2. Case Description

An 11-year-old spayed female Yorkshire Terrier weighing 1.8 kg was presented with a history of chronic left pelvic limb lameness. The dog had undergone surgical correction of a grade III/IV MPL 6 months previously. During that surgery, the tibial tuberosity fragmented while attempting to perform a tibial tuberosity transposition. Fragmentation was sufficient to preclude reattachment of the patella ligament to the proximal tibia. An attempt was made to suture the distal portion of the patella ligament to the tibial crest using an absorbable 2-0 polydioxanone suture (PDS plus, Ethicon, Raritan, NJ, USA). Following surgery, the dog was unable to effectively extend the affected stifle or support weight on the limb.

On physical examination, the dog could not support weight on the left pelvic limb and maintained the limb in a flexed posture. The thigh girth of the affected limb was decreased by 20% compared to the contralateral pelvic limb. A patellar reflex could not be elicited in the left pelvic limb. Cranial drawer and cranial tibial thrust were negative in both stifles. Radiographs of the left stifle revealed proximomedial displacement of the patella relative to the femoral trochlear groove, consistent with patella alta and the absence of the normal protuberance of the tibial tuberosity (Figure 1).

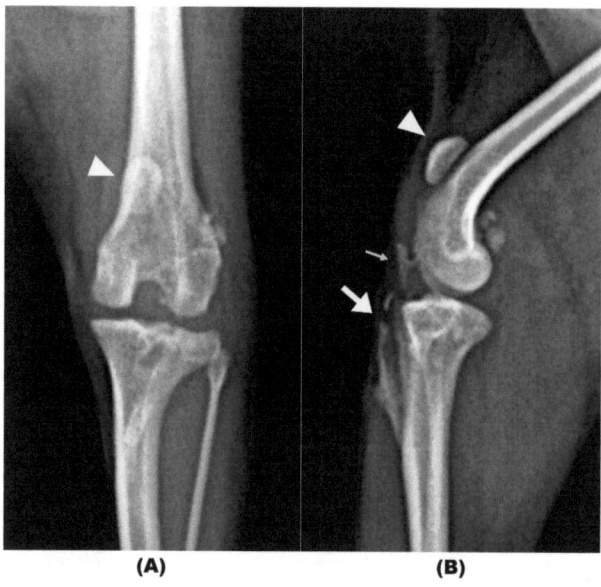

Figure 1. (**A**) Craniocaudal and (**B**) mediolateral radiographic views of the left stifle taken six months following initial surgery to address a grade III/IV medial patellar luxation. The images display tibial tuberosity absorption (white arrow) and proximal dislocation of the patella (arrowhead). Additionally, an ossicle (approximately 5 mm × 1.5 mm) with reduced bone density cranial to the infrapatellar fat pad was observed (yellow arrow).

Surgery involving implantation of a calcaneal tendon–bone allograft to restore the quadriceps extensor mechanism was planned (Figure 2). Tissues had been previously aseptically harvested, with the owner's consent, from a 3-year-old, 4 kg, spayed female mongrel dog euthanized after sustaining a cervical vertebral fracture. The calcaneal tendon included the tendons of the superficial digital flexor, gastrocnemius, and the conjoined tendons from the gracilis, semitendinosus, and biceps femoris muscles and an attached 5 mm × 12 mm bone block were harvested from the calcaneal tuberosity. The tissues were packaged in a sterile container with an antibiotic solution consisting of gentamicin (200 µg/mL), vancomycin (100 µg/mL), and meropenem (200 µg/mL) [17]. The sterile container was sealed within an additional sterile plastic enclosure and frozen at −70 °C. The time from harvesting until use was 4 months. In preparation for implantation, the allograft was thawed in 37 °C sterile physiological saline for 30 min and small pieces of the tendon and bone were excised and submitted for bacterial culture to document that the graft had not been contaminated during the storage period.

The dog was premedicated with hydromorphone (0.1 mg/kg intravenously [IV]) and midazolam (0.2 mg/kg IV). Anesthesia was induced with propofol (4 mg/kg IV) and maintained with 1.5% isoflurane in oxygen. Cefazolin sodium (22 mg/kg IV) was administered 30 min before skin incision and every 90 min during surgery. Intraoperative analgesia was provided using remifentanil (0.1–0.3 µg/kg/min constant rate infusion). A lateral parapatellar approach to the left stifle and proximal tibia was performed [18]. Fibrosis extended cranioproximal from the tibial crest to the distal stump of patellar ligament. A single 5 mm × 1.5 mm bone fragment was visible on the preoperative radiographs and presumed to be a remnant of the tibial tuberosity, but it could not be identified during surgery. After debridement of adherent fibrous tissue, there was an approximately 15 mm gap between the distal end of the patella ligament and the proximal extent of the tibial crest when the stifle was placed in an extended position (Figure 3A). The end of the distal patellar ligament could not be sufficiently mobilized to reattach to the tibia. A lateral parapatellar arthrotomy and medial retinacular release were performed. The cruciate ligaments were intact, and the trochlear groove had sufficient depth to maintain reduction of the patella. The cranioproximal surface of the tibial crest was debrided using a pneumatic burr to remove the granulation tissue which was adhered to the bone. A 0.7 mm Kirschner wire was used to create several holes in the debrided bone bed to expose bleeding cancellous bone. Recombinant human bone morphogenetic protein-2 (rhBMP-2) with hydroxyapatite (HA) (NOVOSIS-Dent, CGBio, Seongnam, Republic of Korea) was placed on the debrided osseous surface (Figure 3B). A mixture of 0.25 mg rhBMP-2 and 0.25 mg of HA was used.

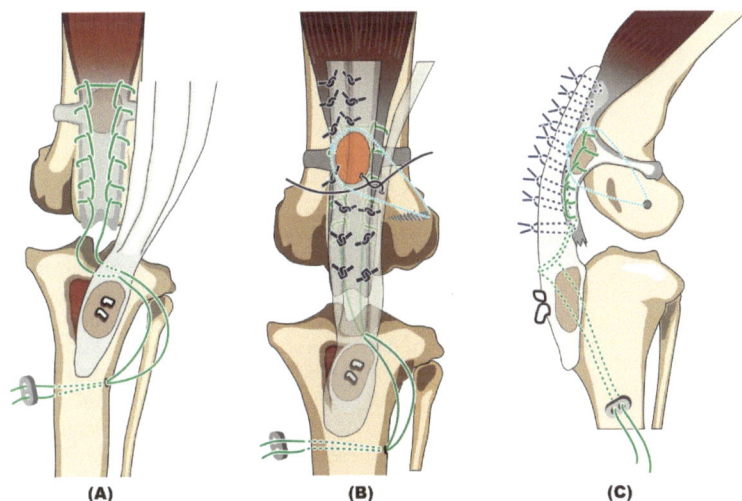

Figure 2. Schematic diagrams illustrating the surgical technique. (**A**) The osseous segment of the calcaneal tendon–bone allograft is secured within the prepared tibial bone bed using two Kirschner wires. A non-absorbable suture is placed through the proximal tibia, patellar ligament, and proximal patellar tendon. (**B**) Craniocaudal and (**C**) mediolateral images show that the allogenic tendon is augmented to enhance both the patellar ligament and the quadriceps tendon. Additionally, an encircling patellar suture is placed as a supplemental restraint to medial luxation.

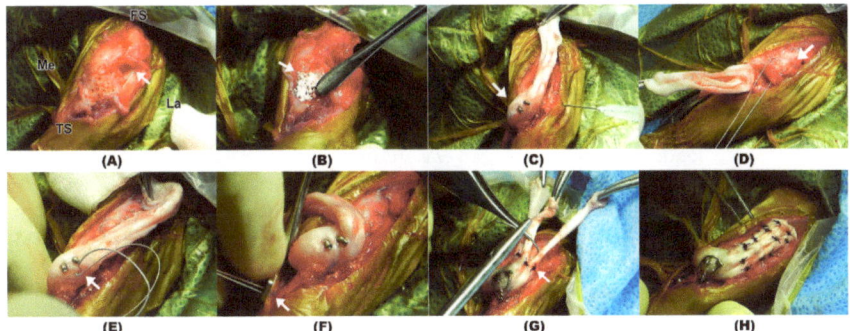

Figure 3. Intraoperative gross photographs. (**A**) Debrided bone displaying multiple holes for osteostixis. A noticeable gap is observed between the distal patellar ligament and the tibial bed (arrow). (**B**) The recombinant human bone morphogenetic protein-2 with hydroxyapatite applied to the bone surface (arrow). (**C**) Allogenic calcaneal bone block secured to the tibial bed using Kirschner wires (arrow). (**D**) A Krackow suture (arrow) initiated at the medial margin of the patellar ligament,

encircling the proximal patella, and terminating at the lateral margin. (**E**) Two free ends of the suture (arrow) exit at the calcaneal bone–tendon allograft junction. (**F**) Both ends of the suture are threaded through the tibia and anchored with a suture button (arrow). (**G**) The grafted tendon is affixed to the patellar ligament and quadriceps tendon using multiple simple interrupted sutures (arrow). (**H**) Gross morphology of the completed implantation of the allograft. FS: femur side; TS: tibia side; Me: medial; La: lateral.

The allograft bone block was secured along the lateral margin of the debrided tibial bone bed using both a 1.1 mm and a 0.9 mm interfragmentary Kirschner wire (Figure 3C). Lateralization of the allogenic bone block established appropriate alignment of the quadriceps mechanism. A strand of multifilament 0 braided non-absorbable suture (FiberWire, Arthrex, Naples, FL, USA) was placed through the proximal tibia, patellar ligament, and proximal patellar tendon to neutralize the force of the quadriceps muscles. Specifically, a Krackow suture pattern was initiated at the distal end of the medial margin of the patellar ligament and continued proximally and passed hemi-circumferentially around the proximal pole of the patella, then coursing distally, with the strand of suture exiting at the distal end of the lateral margin of the patellar ligament (Figure 3D). The two free ends of the suture, emerging from the medial and lateral margins of the distal patellar ligament, passed from the interior to the exterior of the graft tendon at the calcaneal bone–tendon allograft junction (Figure 3E). A transverse bone tunnel was subsequently created through the crainoproximal aspect of the proximal tibia using a 1.4 mm Kirschner wire, and the two free ends of the suture strands were threaded through this tunnel. The suture strands were tensioned to align the patella normally within the trochlear groove, with the stifle positioned at 135° of extension, and the strands were secured through a suture button, and a series of square knots were tied (Figure 3F). A strand of 21-gauge orthopedic wire was placed in a figure-of-eight pattern around the protruding ends of the two interfragmentary Kirschner wires and a transverse hole drilled through the tibia subjacent to the tibial crest, to prevent avulsion of the allograft bone block (Figure 3G). The lateral parapatellar arthrotomy was closed using simple interrupted sutures with 4-0 PDS. To further mitigate the potential of the patella to luxation medially, a suture anchor with a 2-0 non-absorbable braided suture (Micro Corkscrew FT with 2-0 FiberWire, Arthrex, Naples, FL, USA) was placed along the caudal border of the lateral femoral condyle and the suture was placed hemi-circumferentially around the patella, passing through the proximal patellar tendon, lateral retinaculum, and distal patellar tendon, and securely tied.

The allogenic calcaneal tendon was trimmed to the appropriate length (4 cm) to cover the patellar ligament and quadriceps tendon. With the stifle positioned in full extension, components of the grafted tendon were individually sutured to the host tissue while maintaining proximal traction on the graft. The allogenic superficial digital flexor tendon was anchored to the patellar ligament and the central portion of the quadriceps tendon using a simple interrupted suture with a 3-0 PDS. The lateral (the conjoined tendon of the gracilis, semitendinosus, and biceps femoris muscles) and medial (the gastrocnemius tendon) flap of the allograft was sutured to the lateral and medial retinaculum, as well as the lateral and medial portions of the quadriceps tendon, respectively, using 3-0 PDS in a simple interrupted suture pattern (Figure 3H). The stifle was placed through a range of motion, and the patella tacked appropriately in the trochlear groove and did not luxate. A swab of the surgical site was obtained for bacterial culture prior to closure. The subcutaneous tissue and skin were closed in a routine manner.

3. Results

On postoperative radiographs, the patella was positioned appropriately in the trochlear groove. The allogenic bone block appeared to be securely attached to the tibia by the Kirschner wires and figure-of-eight wire (Figure 4). The postoperative patellar ligament length (PLL) to the patella length (PL) ratio in the left stifle was calculated to be 1.42, which was similar to a 1.41 PLL:PL ratio calculated on a radiograph of the contralateral stifle which was obtained postoperatively [19]. Following surgery, the dog was administered cephalexin (22 mg/kg PO, two times daily) for 1 week and carprofen (2.2 mg/kg PO, two times daily) for 2 weeks. The limb was immobilized in a modified Robert Jones bandage, and the dog was confined to a cage for 2 weeks.

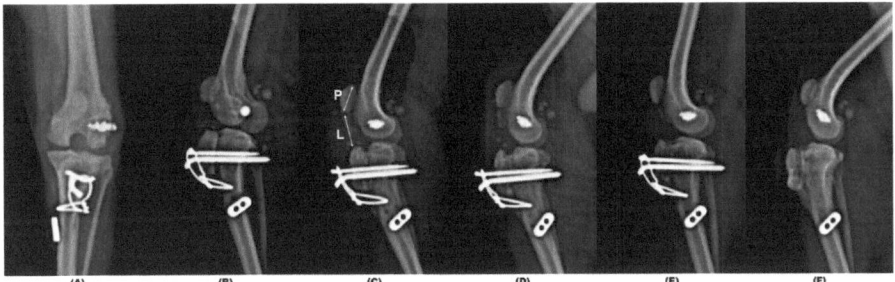

Figure 4. Immediate postoperative craniocaudal (**A**) and mediolateral (**B**) radiographic images, alongside sequential postoperative mediolateral radiographic images at immediate (**C**), 4 weeks (**D**), 12 weeks (**E**), and 28 weeks (**F**) post-surgery, with a PLL (marked as L in (**C**)): PL (marked as P in (**C**)) of 1.42, 1.46, 1.54 and 1.54, respectively. The patella remains normally positioned within the trochlear groove across all stages. The reconstruction of the tibial tuberosity using a calcaneus bone block allograft is distinctly visible. Due to skin irritation caused by the protruding ends of the Kirschner wires, pins and tension band wiring were removed at 26 weeks post-surgery. PLL, patellar ligament length; PL, patella length.

The dog was re-evaluated 2 weeks following surgery, and the incision had healed without complications. The dog was able to bear weight on the involved limb while standing and had a mild weight-bearing lameness with a decreased range of motion in the left stifle. Cultures of the allograft tendon and the surgical site obtained prior to closure had not yielded bacterial growth. Cage confinement was continued for an additional 2 weeks without bandaging the limb. Two weeks postoperatively, by 4 weeks postoperatively, the dog still had a mild weight-bearing lameness, and the owners were allowed to institute slow walks on a leash for 5–10 min twice daily; the duration of these walks was gradually increased to 30 min over 12 weeks. Both passive range of motion exercises and thermotherapy were also initiated twice daily at 4 weeks and continued until 12 weeks. The dog was re-evaluated 12 weeks following surgery. The dog had a weight-bearing lameness but could freely extend the right stifle with a near-normal range of motion in the joint. Radiographs obtained at 12 weeks revealed that interface between the grafted bone and the host bone could no longer be defined, and the patella continued to be properly positioned in the trochlear groove. Ultrasonography was performed 6 months postoperatively which revealed homogeneous continuity of the reconstructed patellar ligament between the grafted bone block and the distal pole of the patella. The Kirschner and tension band wires were removed 6 months following surgery as the protruding ends of the Kirschner wires were causing irritation of the overlying skin. By 7 months postoperatively, the dog was perceived to have a normal gait, and the patella was stable during manipulation. The dog could jump on and off a couch, although the thigh girth of the left pelvic limb was approximately 7% less than that of the unaffected limb. The left PLL:PL ratio had increased slightly to 1.54. The owner reported via telephone that the dog effectively used the left pelvic limb without lameness until the dog died of degenerative mitral valve disease 29 months after the surgery.

4. Discussion

A composite calcaneal tendon–bone block allograft was utilized to effectively restore the quadriceps extensor mechanism in the dog in the current case report. Reattachment of the patella ligament to the tibia in the dog described in this case report was complicated by resorption of the fragmented tibial tuberosity and extensive parenchymal loss of the distal patella ligament. Simple tenorrhaphy was not a viable treatment option due to the loss of the distal portion of the patellar ligament and the absence of the tibial tuberosity [20,21]. Additionally, direct attachment of the distal patellar ligament to the tibial bone seemed impractical due to a larger anticipated gap resulting from chronic quadriceps tendon contraction and debridement of the distal patellar ligament stump. Even if ligament-to-bone fixation were feasible, the repair would need to be protected for an extended period of time, given that ligament-to-bone healing typically progresses slower than ligament-to-ligament healing [22]. Therefore, any tenorrhaphy repair technique employed would have been unlikely to withstand the increased tension during surgery and the postoperative convalescent period [22]. Given these challenges, we elected to employ a novel surgical approach to effectively restore the function of the quadriceps extensor mechanism.

In assessing surgical strategies to bridge the gap between the remaining proximal portion of the patella ligament and an insertion point on the proximal tibia, we contemplated the use of either an isolated autogenous or allogenic tendon graft. Given the degree of tension the quadriceps mechanism would exert on any repair technique, we had concerns that the sutures placed at the graft–patellar ligament interface might dehisce and even greater concerns for dehiscence where the graft would be secured to the proximal tibia. The tendon graft-to-bone healing process involves multiple stages, including the development of fibrovascular interface tissue, gradual mineralization, and the penetration of bone into the outer layer of the grafted tendon [23]. Consequently, the time required for tendon graft-to-bone healing is typically longer compared to the relatively straightforward process of tendon-bone graft-to-bone healing, which involves direct bone growth and remodeling [23]. In addition, a previous study demonstrated that the bone-to-bone interface was superior to the bone–tendon interface in terms of mechanical strength, as indicated by higher failure stress [24]. Another in vivo comparative study recommended reconstructing the bone–tendon insertion interface by repairing between homogenous tissues [25]. Furthermore, studies have demonstrated that the integration of grafted tendon into host bone is slower and more susceptible to fixation failure compared to the integration of the host–graft osseous interface when using a composite tendon–bone allograft [16,17]. Additionally, there were concerns regarding abnormal biomechanical stress being placed on the patellofemoral articulation if we secured the patellar ligament in a caudal location due to loss of this dog's tibial tuberosity, which might also contribute to dehiscence or hinder an optimal return to function [26–28].

These factors steered us to consider using a composite tendon–bone graft in this dog. Experimental studies in rabbits and clinical applications in human patients have reported strong, long-term integration at the graft–host osseous bone interface following implantation of allogenic composite tendon–bone grafts [29,30]. We felt that a composite tendon–bone graft would afford a secure means of performing a tenorrhaphy, provide reliable fixation of the ligament to the tibia, and contribute to the reconstruction of the normal morphology of the tibial tuberosity. In this case, an allograft was selected instead of an autograft to circumvent issues harvesting a suitable tendon–bone graft, which is particularly problematic in a toy breed dog. The use of an allograft eliminated any risks associated with donor site morbidity and the potential for extended surgical time associated with harvesting the graft [10,29]. Despite numerous studies reporting successful outcomes with bone–tendon allografts [6,12,13], concerns remain regarding infection, immune-mediated rejection, and the potential for nonunion or delayed union of the grafted bone segment [31,32]. In this case, the recipient bone bed consisted predominantly of cortical bone, with little exposed cancellous bone, which prompted our use of rhBMP-2 with HA to promote osseous union. The use of rhBMP-2 and HA has been shown to increase vascularization and osseous integration of cortical bone allografts [33]. Fortunately, there were no overt clinical or radiographic abnormalities suggestive of infection or immune rejection in the dog reported here. Caution is, however, advised when employing such allografts, as asepsis needs to be immaculate to prevent infection and the graft must be processed appropriately to mitigate the host's immune response [31,32].

The allogenic bone block was positioned and secured along the lateral margin of the debrided tibial bone bed to the alignment of the quadriceps mechanism. An encircling patellar suture was placed and secured to the caudolateral femoral condyle as a supplemental restraint to medial luxation [34,35]. Patella luxation was never observed or elicited following surgery.

After tenorrhaphy, it is imperative to maintain apposition of the tendon ends, or the tendon-to-bone interface, without gap formation until the healing process is complete [36–38]. A gap exceeding 3 mm between the apposed surfaces has been shown to reduce tensile strength and lead to suboptimal functional outcomes [36]. Relying solely on suture techniques has been shown to be inadequate in preventing gap formation throughout the healing phase of the postoperative convalescent period [37,38]. Consequently, supplemental stabilization methods are often utilized to protect tenorrhaphies during the initial postoperative convalescent period [38]. Placement of a trans-articular external fixator has been advocated to immobilize the stifle and to mitigate tensile forces exerted by the quadriceps muscles following patella tendon repair [38,39]. A fixator was not utilized in the dog in this case report because the dog's weight was <2 kg. Fixators provide greater stability and are easier to apply and manage in large dogs and the risk of fracture through one of the pin tracks is a valid concern in small toy breed dogs [40,41]. A robust suture was placed, which engaged the proximal pole of the patella and secured to the proximal tibia, to mitigate tension on the repair in this dog. A similar supplement suture technique was shown to enhance biomechanical properties following primary patella ligament repair in a human cadaveric study [42]. Additionally, individual components of the allograft tendon were draped over the patella ligament and quadriceps tendon and secured to those structures using on-lay suturing, rather than performing a simple end-to-end tenorrhaphy. This method of augmented allogenic tendon repair yields immediate enhancement in the mechanical properties of the repair, surpassing those of primary tenorrhaphy alone [43]. During the suturing of the grafted tendon to the host tendon, the allografted tendon was tensioned while the stifle was maintained in full extension. This technique is supported by the results reported in a retrospective study, which found that successful restoration of the knee extensor mechanism is more likely when the allograft is tensioned rather than loosely attached during suturing in human patients with chronic patellar rupture [13].

This technique may be applied to chronic damage of the tendon–bone interface, such as the triceps brachii tendon–olecranon tuber and Achilles tendon–calcaneal tuberosity, when the tendons are completely transected and shortened, or the bony prominences are reabsorbed, making reconstruction between homogenous tissues difficult. For broader application of this technique, further study regarding in vivo biomechanical and histological examination would be necessary. There are several limitations to this technique, including difficulties in acquiring and storing the allograft, size differences between the graft and the host bed, and potential host responses to the allograft. Additionally, this study has limitations, as it is a single case report without biomechanical testing prior to application.

5. Conclusions

The tendon–bone allograft was particularly useful in the dog reported here because of the dog's abnormal tibial tuberosity morphology. This surgical technique would appear to be applicable in analogous cases involving irreparable tibial avulsion fractures, when there is extensive patellar tendon loss or a primary tenorrhaphy is unlikely to be successful; however, further validation of this surgical technique through cadaveric studies and additional clinical trials is essential.

Author Contributions: Conceptualization, H.L., D.D.L., J.J. and Y.J.; methodology, H.K., H.L. and Y.J.; software, H.K., J.J., G.K. and Y.J.; validation, H.L., D.D.L., J.J. and Y.J.; formal analysis, H.K., H.L. and J.J.; investigation, H.K., H.L., D.D.L., J.J. and G.K.; resources, H.L., J.J. and Y.J.; data curation, H.K., H.L. and Y.J.X; writing—original draft preparation, H.K. and H.L.; writing—review and editing,

D.D.L., J.J. and Y.J.; visualization, H.K., H.L., J.J. and G.K.; supervision, H.L., D.D.L., J.J. and Y.J.; project administration, H.L., J.J. and Y.J.; funding acquisition, H.L. All authors have read and agreed to the published version of the manuscript.

Funding: This research was supported by a basic science research program through the National Research Foundation of Korea (NRF) funded by the Ministry of Education (RS-2023-00247989).

Institutional Review Board Statement: Ethical review and approval were not required as we report a case study from a veterinary hospital. We have the consent of both the owner and veterinarian that this dog (underwent the listed examinations and surgical intervention) was treated not for an experimental but for a medical reason.

Informed Consent Statement: The patient was a client-owned animal and written informed consent was obtained from the owner of the animal.

Data Availability Statement: The data presented in this study are available on justified request from the corresponding author.

Conflicts of Interest: The authors declare no conflicts of interest.

References

1. Cashmore, R.; Havlicek, M.; Perkins, N.; James, D.; Fearnside, S.; Marchevsky, A.; Black, A. Major complications and risk factors associated with surgical correction of congenital medial patellar luxation in 124 dogs. *Vet. Comp. Orthop. Traumatol.* **2014**, *27*, 263–270. [CrossRef] [PubMed]
2. Oshin, A. Complications associated with the treatment of patellar luxation. In *Complications in Small Animal Surgery*; Griffon, D., Hamaide, A., Eds.; Wiley Blackwell: Hoboken, NJ, USA, 2016; pp. 889–896.
3. Cofone, M.; Smith, G.; Lenehan, T.; Newton, C. Unilateral and bilateral stifle arthrodesis in eight dogs. *Vet. Surg.* **1992**, *21*, 299–303. [CrossRef] [PubMed]
4. James, R.; Kesturu, G.; Balian, G.; Chhabra, A.B. Tendon: Biology, biomechanics, repair, growth factors, and evolving treatment options. *J. Hand Surg.* **2008**, *33*, 102–112. [CrossRef]
5. King, C.M.; Vartivarian, M. Achilles tendon rupture repair: Simple to complex. *Clin. Podiatr. Med. Sur* **2023**, *40*, 75–96. [CrossRef] [PubMed]
6. Song, I.; Ngan, A. Reconstruction of an Achilles rupture with 12 cm defect utilizing Achilles tendon allograft and calcaneal bone block: A case report. *Foot Ankle Online J.* **2020**, *13*, 11.
7. Hanna, T.; Dripchak, P.; Childress, T. Chronic Achilles rupture repair by allograft with bone block fixation: Technique tip. *Foot Ankle Int.* **2014**, *35*, 168–174. [CrossRef] [PubMed]
8. Jiménez-Carrasco, C.; Ammari-Sánchez-Villanueva, F.; Prada-Chamorro, E.; García-Guirao, A.J.; Tejero, S. Allograft and autologous reconstruction techniques for neglected achilles tendon rupture: A mid-long-term follow-up analysis. *J. Clin. Med.* **2023**, *12*, 1135. [CrossRef]
9. Farrell, M.; Fitzpatrick, N. Patellar ligament-bone autograft for reconstruction of a distal patellar ligament defect in a dog. *J. Small Anim. Pract.* **2013**, *54*, 269–274. [CrossRef]
10. Grove, J.R.; Hardy, M.A. Autograft, allograft and xenograft options in the treatment of neglected Achilles tendon ruptures: A historical review with illustration of surgical repair. *Foot Ankle J.* **2008**, *1*, 1. [CrossRef]
11. Sanchez-Sotelo, J.; Morrey, B.F.; Adams, R.A.; O'Driscoll, S.W. Reconstruction of chronic ruptures of the distal biceps tendon with use of an achilles tendon allograft. *J. Bone Jt. Surg.* **2002**, *84*, 999–1005. [CrossRef] [PubMed]
12. Burnett, R.S.; Butler, R.; Barrack, R. Extensor mechanism allograft reconstruction in TKA at a mean of 56 months. *Clin. Orthop. Relat. Res.* **2006**, *452*, 159–165. [CrossRef] [PubMed]
13. Burnett, R.S.J.; Berger, R.A.; Paprosky, W.G.; Della Valle, C.J.; Jacobs, J.J.; Rosenberg, A.G. Extensor mechanism allograft reconstruction after total knee arthroplasty: A comparison of two techniques. *J. Bone Jt. Surg.* **2004**, *86*, 2694–2699. [CrossRef] [PubMed]
14. Dandu, N.; Trasolini, N.A.; DeFroda, S.F.; Holland, T.; Yanke, A.B. Revision quadriceps tendon repair with bone-Achilles allograft augmentation. *Video J. Sports Med.* **2021**, *1*, 26350254211032680. [CrossRef]
15. Alam, M.; Gordon, W.; Heo, S.; Lee, K.; Kim, N.; Kim, M.; Lee, H. Augmentation of ruptured tendon using fresh frozen Achilles tendon allograft in two dogs: A case report. *Vet. Med.* **2013**, *58*, 50–55. [CrossRef]
16. Serra, C.I.; Navarro, P.; Guillem, R.; Soler, C. Use of frozen tendon allograft in two clinical cases: Common calcaneal tendon and patellar ligament rupture. *J. Am. Anim. Hosp. Assoc.* **2020**, *56*, 315. [CrossRef] [PubMed]
17. Paolin, A.; Spagnol, L.; Battistella, G.; Trojan, D. Evaluation of allograft decontamination with two different antibiotic cocktails at the Treviso Tissue Bank Foundation. *PLoS ONE* **2018**, *13*, e0201792. [CrossRef] [PubMed]
18. Johnson, K.A. Approach to the stifle joint through a lateral incision. In *Piermattei's Atlas of Surgical Approaches to the Bones and Joints of the Dog and Cat, 5 ed.*; Elsevier Saunders Missouri: St. Louis, MO, USA, 2014; pp. 392–395.

19. Johnson, A.L.; Broaddus, K.D.; Hauptman, J.G.; Marsh, S.; Monsere, J.; Sepulveda, G. Vertical patellar position in large-breed dogs with clinically normal stifles and large-breed dogs with medial patellar luxation. *Vet. Surg.* **2006**, *35*, 78–81. [CrossRef] [PubMed]
20. Magnussen, R.A.; Lustig, S.; Demey, G.; Masdar, H.; ElGuindy, A.; Servien, E.; Neyret, P. Reconstruction of chronic patellar tendon ruptures with extensor mechanism allograft. *Tech. Knee Surg.* **2012**, *11*, 34–40. [CrossRef]
21. Panagopoulos, A.; Antzoulas, P.; Giakoumakis, S.; Konstantopoulou, A.; Tagaris, G. Neglected rupture of the patellar tendon after fixation of tibial tubercle avulsion in an adolescent male managed with ipsilateral semitendinosus autograft reconstruction. *Cureus* **2021**, *13*, e15368. [CrossRef] [PubMed]
22. Weiler, A.; Scheffler, S.; Apreleva, M. Healing of ligament and tendon to bone. In *Repair and Regeneration of Ligaments, Tendons and Joint Capsule*; Walsh, W.R., Ed.; Humana Press Inc.: Totowa, NJ, USA, 2006; pp. 201–232.
23. Ekdahl, M.; Wang, J.H.-C.; Ronga, M.; Fu, F.H. Graft healing in anterior cruciate ligament reconstruction. *Knee Surg. Sports Traumatol. Arthrosc.* **2008**, *16*, 935–947. [CrossRef] [PubMed]
24. Leung, K.S.; Qin, L.; Fu, L.K.; Chan, C.W. A comparative study of bone to bone repair and bone to tendon healing in patella–patellar tendon complex in rabbits. *Clin. Biomech.* **2002**, *17*, 594–602. [CrossRef] [PubMed]
25. Leung, K.S.; Chong, W.S.; Chow, D.H.K.; Zhang, P.; Cheung, W.H.; Wong, M.W.N.; Qin, L. A comparative study on the biomechanical and histological properties of bone-to-bone, bone-to-tendon, and tendon-to-tendon healing: An Achilles tendon–calcaneus model in goats. *Am. J. Sports Med.* **2015**, *43*, 1413–1421. [CrossRef] [PubMed]
26. Atzmon, R.; Steen, A.; Vel, M.S.; Pierre, K.; Murray, I.R.; Sherman, S.L. Tibial tubercle osteotomy to unload the patellofemoral joint. *J. Cartil. Jt. Preserv.* **2023**, *3*, 100112. [CrossRef]
27. Park, D.; Kang, J.; Kim, N.; Heo, S. Patellofemoral contact mechanics after transposition of tibial tuberosity in dogs. *J. Vet. Sci.* **2020**, *21*, e67. [CrossRef] [PubMed]
28. Yoo, Y.-H.; Lee, S.-J.; Jeong, S.-W. Effects of quadriceps angle on patellofemoral contact pressure. *J. Vet. Sci.* **2020**, *21*, e69. [CrossRef]
29. Chen, G.; Zhang, H.; Ma, Q.; Zhao, J.; Zhang, Y.; Fan, Q.; Ma, B. Fresh-frozen complete extensor mechanism allograft versus autograft reconstruction in rabbits. *Sci. Rep.* **2016**, *6*, 22106. [CrossRef] [PubMed]
30. Olson, E.J.; Harner, C.D.; Fu, F.H.; Silbey, M.B. Clinical use of fresh, frozen soft tissue allografts. *Orthopedics* **1992**, *15*, 1225–1232. [CrossRef] [PubMed]
31. Barrios, R.; Leyes, M.; Amillo, S.; Oteiza, C. Bacterial contamination of allografts. *Acta Orthop. Belg.* **1994**, *60*, 152. [PubMed]
32. Garbuz, D.S.; Masri, B.A.; Czitrom, A.A. Biology of allografting. *Orthop. Clin. N. Am.* **1998**, *29*, 199–204. [CrossRef] [PubMed]
33. Pluhar, G.E.; Manley, P.A.; Heiner, J.P.; Vanderby, R., Jr.; Seeherman, H.J.; Markel, M.D. The effect of recombinant human bone morphogenetic protein-2 on femoral reconstruction with an intercalary allograft in a dog model. *J. Orthop. Res.* **2001**, *19*, 308–317. [CrossRef] [PubMed]
34. Choi, H.; Kim, S.; Han, C.; Jang, A.; Jung, H.; Hwang, T.; Lee, H.; Hwang, Y.; Lee, W.; Lee, S. Surgical correction of medial patellar luxation including release of vastus median's without trochleoplasty in small breed dogs: A retrospective review of 22 cases. *J. Vet. Clin.* **2018**, *35*, 71–76. [CrossRef]
35. Mazdarani, P.; Miles, J.E. Ideal anchor points for patellar anti-rotational sutures for management of medial patellar luxation in dogs: A radiographic survey. *Vet. Comp. Orthop. Traumatol.* **2023**, *36*, 068–074. [CrossRef]
36. Gelberman, R.H.; Boyer, M.I.; Brodt, M.D.; Winters, S.C.; Silva, M.J. The effect of gap formation at the repair site on the strength and excursion of intrasynovial flexor tendons. An experimental study on the early stages of tendon-healing in dogs. *J. Bone Jt. Surg.* **1999**, *81*, 975–982. [CrossRef] [PubMed]
37. Moores, A.P.; Comerford, E.J.; Tarlton, J.F.; Owen, M.R. Biomechanical and clinical evaluation of a modified 3-loop pulley suture pattern for reattachment of canine tendons to bone. *Vet. Surg.* **2004**, *33*, 391–397. [CrossRef] [PubMed]
38. Tidwell, S.J.; Greenwood, K.; Franklin, S.P. Novel Achilles tendon repair technique utilizing an allograft and hybrid external fixator in dogs. *Open Vet. J.* **2022**, *12*, 335–340. [CrossRef] [PubMed]
39. Tidwell, S.J.; Franklin, S.P. Patellar tendon repair using a patellar tendon allograft and external fixator in three dogs. *VCOT Open* **2022**, *5*, e98–e102. [CrossRef]
40. Bakici, M.; Karslı, B.; Cebeci, M.T. External skeletal fixation. *Int. J. Vet. Anim. Res.* **2019**, *2*, 69–73.
41. Knudsen, C.; Arthurs, G.; Hayes, G.; Langley-Hobbs, S. Long bone fracture as a complication following external skeletal fixation: 11 cases. *J. Small Anim. Pract.* **2012**, *53*, 687–692. [CrossRef] [PubMed]
42. Gehrmann, R.; Harten, R.; Renard, R.; Rao, J.; Spencer, J. Biomechanical evaluation of patellar tendon repair techniques: Comparison of double Krackow stitch with and without cerclage augmentation. *MOJ Orthop. Rheumatol.* **2016**, *5*, 00163. [CrossRef]
43. Barber, F.A.; McGarry, J.E.; Herbert, M.A.; Anderson, R.B. A biomechanical study of Achilles tendon repair augmentation using GraftJacket matrix. *Foot Ankle Int.* **2008**, *29*, 329–333. [CrossRef] [PubMed]

Disclaimer/Publisher's Note: The statements, opinions and data contained in all publications are solely those of the individual author(s) and contributor(s) and not of MDPI and/or the editor(s). MDPI and/or the editor(s) disclaim responsibility for any injury to people or property resulting from any ideas, methods, instructions or products referred to in the content.

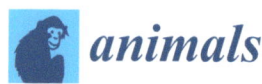

Article

Knee Joint Osteoarthritis in Overweight Cats: The Clinical and Radiographic Findings

Joanna Bonecka [1,*], Michał Skibniewski [2], Paweł Zep [3] and Małgorzata Domino [4,*]

[1] Department of Small Animal Diseases and Clinic, Institute of Veterinary Medicine, Warsaw University of Life Sciences (WULS-SGGW), 02-787 Warsaw, Poland
[2] Department of Morphological Sciences, Institute of Veterinary Medicine, Warsaw University of Life Sciences (WULS-SGGW), 02-787 Warsaw, Poland; michal_skibniewski@sggw.edu.pl
[3] OchWET Veterinary Clinic, 02-119 Warszawa, Poland; pawel.zep@ochwet.pl
[4] Department of Large Animal Diseases and Clinic, Institute of Veterinary Medicine, Warsaw University of Life Sciences (WULS-SGGW), 02-787 Warsaw, Poland
* Correspondence: joanna_bonecka@sggw.edu.pl (J.B.); malgorzata_domino@sggw.edu.pl (M.D.); Tel.: +48-22-59-36-174 (J.B.); +48-22-59-36-191 (M.D.)

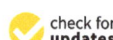

Citation: Bonecka, J.; Skibniewski, M.; Zep, P.; Domino, M. Knee Joint Osteoarthritis in Overweight Cats: The Clinical and Radiographic Findings. *Animals* **2023**, *13*, 2427. https://doi.org/10.3390/ani13152427

Academic Editors: L. Miguel Carreira and João Alves

Received: 29 June 2023
Revised: 21 July 2023
Accepted: 25 July 2023
Published: 27 July 2023

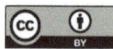

Copyright: © 2023 by the authors. Licensee MDPI, Basel, Switzerland. This article is an open access article distributed under the terms and conditions of the Creative Commons Attribution (CC BY) license (https:// creativecommons.org/licenses/by/ 4.0/).

Simple Summary: Osteoarthritis (OA) is a common condition among cats. It is characterized by progressive degenerative joint disease. OA results from repair and degeneration of articular cartilage, in association with alterations in subchondral bone metabolism, osteophytosis, and synovial inflammation. In cats, OA is often secondary to an underlying cause, such as trauma. Cats with knee joint OA can show typical symptoms including a general reduction in activity, reluctance to jump, deterioration in appearance, and even aggression. Subtle symptoms that owners can observe are reluctance to move and apathy. Cats with knee problems may not show the typical clinical symptoms of lameness. After excluding other causes of disturbing symptoms, further diagnostic imaging is advised to visualize typical radiographic signs of OA. Thus, visualization of osteophytes, enthesophytes, effusion, soft tissue swelling, subchondral sclerosis, and intra-articular mineralization can be used to score the severity of OA. This study aimed to investigate the occurrence of clinical symptoms and radiological signs of knee joint OA in cats and to assess their prevalence concerning cats' body condition scores. Radiographic imaging of the knee joints of 64 cats was performed, and considered signs were compared between underweight, normal-weight, and overweight groups. Severe feline knee joint OA appears with similar frequency in underweight, normal-weight, and overweight cats. Therefore, regardless of the cat's body weight, when the owner reports any unusual behavior of the cat, the veterinarian should take a detailed history driven to identify non-specific clinical symptoms of OA.

Abstract: Despite a high prevalence of osteoarthritis (OA) reported in the domesticated cat population, studies on feline knee joint OA are scarcer. Knee joint OA is a painful, age-related, chronic degenerative joint disease that significantly affects cats' activity and quality of life. In dogs and humans, one may consider overweight as a risk factor for the development and progression of knee joint OA; therefore, this study aims to assess the severity of knee joint OA in the body-weight-related groups of cats concerning clinical symptoms and radiographic signs. The study was conducted on sixty-four ($n = 64$) cats with confirmed OA. The demographic data on sex, neutering, age, and breed were collected. Then, the body condition score (BCS) was assessed, and each cat was allocated to the underweight, normal-weight, or overweight group. Within clinical symptoms, joint pain, joint swelling, joint deformities, lameness, reluctance to move, and apathy were graded. Based on the radiographic signs, minor OA, mild OA, moderate OA, and severe OA were scored. Prevalence and co-occurrence of the studied variables were then assessed. Joint pain was elicited in 20–31% of the OA-affected joints, joint deformities in 21–30%, and lameness in 20–54%, with no differences between weight-related groups. Severe OA was detected in 10–16% of the OA-affected joints, with no differences between weight-related groups. Severe OA in feline knee joints appears with similar frequency in overweight, underweight, and normal-weight cats. However, the general prevalence of clinical symptoms and radiographic signs is different in overweight cats.

Keywords: BCS; radiographic signs; severity; radiographs; feline

1. Introduction

The Osteoarthritis Research Society International (OARSI) defined osteoarthritis (OA) as a disorder affecting movable joints that manifests first as an abnormal joint tissue metabolism and next as functional derangements often leading to illness [1]. Thus, OA is considered as a common chronic degenerative form of arthritis that affects the synovial joints of humans and various species of animals [2,3]. The prevalence of OA in cats ranges from 16% to 91% [4–9], depending on the studied population. Clarke et al. [4] reported a 16% prevalence of OA in a population of 218 cats, aged from 0.2 to 18 years. Godfrey [5] showed a 22% prevalence of OA in a population of 491 cats, aged from 3 to 19 years. Hardie et al. [6] reported a 26% prevalence of appendicula joint OA in a population of 100 cats older than 12 years. Freire et al. [7] evidenced a 46% prevalence of appendicula OA in a group of 30 cats at an average age of 12 years. Slingerland et al. [8] showed a 61% prevalence of OA in a population of 100 cats older than 6 years but only 5% in knee joints. Finally, Lascelles et al. [9] noted a 91% prevalence of OA in a similar population of 100 cats, where knee joint OA was reported in 50% of affected joint OA [9]. As the prevalence of feline OA increased with age [9], currently the cat's age is considered to be an identified OA risk factor [8,9].

Considering feline OA etiology, primary and secondary OA are distinguished. The term primary OA is used for idiopathic OA in Scottish Fold affected by osteochondrodysplasia [10] or mucopolysaccharidosis [11]. The majority of cases of primary OA have no identified initiating factor and are referred to as age-related cartilage degeneration seen in older cats [9]. On the other hand, secondary OA may be caused by congenital joint malformation, joint deformity, joint dislocation, traumatic joint injury, and hypervitaminosis A [9,12,13]. It may develop as a consequence of hip dysplasia in susceptible breeds [14,15], patellar luxation in more susceptible Abyssinian and Devon Rex cats [16–18], or patellar displacement, which is more common in Domestic Shorthair cats [19]. Moreover, secondary OA may appear after joint infection, as in the case of *Mycoplasma* spp. infection in polyarthritis [13], as well as after nonspecific infection when the immune response is defective [20].

One should consider that the etiology and the mechanism underlying the pathogenesis of OA are not fully understood; therefore, the treatment is focused on reducing clinical symptoms and if possible disease-modifying therapies [21]. Unlike dogs, whose lameness is the major clinical symptom of OA [22], clinical symptoms of feline OA are subtle [23,24]. Among them, the stress response is clinically the most difficult manifestation of chronic pain to recognize. The clinical symptoms of feline OA include apathy, joint pain on palpation, joint swelling, joint deformities, impaired function of the affected joint manifested by lameness, and reluctance to move [5–7,13,25–28]. Thus, the symptom-reducing therapy in cats is based on the administration of non-steroidal anti-inflammatory drugs (NSAIDs). However, their use in cats with stable renal insufficiency has potential drawbacks such as a higher level of proteinuria [29]. Meloxicam is the most popular, long-term, safe NSAID prescribed by veterinary surgeons and orthopedists [30]. Another NSAID, robenacoxib, is a highly selective COX-2 inhibitor developed as a painkiller and anti-inflammatory drug for dogs and cats, which can be used without adverse effects [31,32]. One may observe that OA pain is more complex than inflammatory pain alone [33]; therefore, an appropriate painkiller targeted at neuropathic pain is occasionally necessary. The study on cats with OA showed that the administration of gabapentin, a gamma-aminobutyric acid (GABA) receptor agonist, improves the cat's activity levels [34]. Another study on old cats with OA demonstrated desirable painkilling outcomes after the administration of tramadol, an opioid receptor agonist [33]. A recent study in 2021, introduced frunevetmab, the feline monoclonal antibody therapy, into the treatment of chronic pain in cats with OA and reported significant improvement in cats' behavior [35,36]. However, one may postulate that cats disguise part of the clinical symptoms of disease due to the instinct for self-preservation [37], due to the solitary and territorial innate behavior of cats. Therefore, the treatment strategy for cats with OA should consider the pharmacological symptom-reducing therapy with anti-inflammatory or analgetic drugs used in combination with joint supplementation, and rehabilitation. Surgery should be considered the last resort [9,28,38,39].

OA manifests itself in cartilage degradation, increase in cartilage cell metabolism, synovial inflammation, hyperplasia, and hypertrophy as well as bone changes, of which bone changes are the most reliably identifiable radiologically [4–6,9,27]. Thus, radiographic imaging enables the diagnosis of OA by exposing the radiographic signs of degenerative changes in the affected joint. Therefore, the use of coherent terminology and standardized nomenclature is necessary for the proper OA recognition and the feasible assessment of disease severity and progression. One may observe that the degenerative changes in the feline knee joints are radiologically characterized by the presence of the narrow and irregular joint space (thin and uneven lucency between the adjacent cortical bones); osteophytes and enthesiophytes (bone outgrowths on the surface of cortical bone); subchondral bone cyst (the osteolytic area of well-delimited increased lucency, localized in the cortical and subcortical bone) and/or subchondral bone sclerosis (the area of increased opacity within the cortical and subcortical bone); periosteal proliferation (the area of mildly increased opacity outside the cortical bone), and intra-articular mineralization (the area of severely increased opacity inside joint space) [4,5,13,15,26,40–43]. Assessment of the particular radiographic signs allows for the determination of disease severity considering the clinical symptoms.

We hypothesized that in the feline knee joint, severe OA is more frequent in overweight than in underweight and normal-weight cats and is associated with more severe clinical symptoms. Thus, the objectives of the present study were: (1) to assess the severity of knee joint OA in the overweight, underweight, and normal-weight groups of cats concerning cats' age and sex; (2) to explore whether overweight is associated with more severe clinical symptoms; (3) to explore whether overweight is associated with OA severity.

2. Materials and Methods

2.1. Study Design

A study was conducted on six hundred and sixty-two (n = 662) cats presented for radiological examination of pelvic limbs. Examinations were performed between 2019 and 2022 in the Small Animal Clinic at the Institute of Veterinary Medicine at the Warsaw University of Life Sciences. All cats represented privately owned clinical patients. Owners provided written consent for the cat's inclusion in the study. All the performed procedures represented the standard diagnostic tests; therefore, no ethical approval was required. The type of the study was categorized as prospective, longitudinal, and observational.

2.2. Clinical Data Collection

All cats underwent an initial examination that included the collection of medical history as well as general physical and detailed orthopedic examinations. In the medical history, data on sex, neutering, age, and breed as well as reluctance to move and apathy were obtained from each cat. The reluctance to move and apathy were assessed by the owner in the cat's own environment. The reluctance to move was considered present when the owner reported that the cat did not want to move even when the owner encouraged the cat to move with a treat. The apathy was considered present when the cat manifested a lack of interest or concern compared to the previous, normal behavior of this cat. Body weight was measured using an electronic scale (Veterinary Scale for small animal practice, Bielskie Wagi, Bielsko-Biala, Poland). The body condition score (BCS) was used to assign cats to groups, as the body weight standard varies between cat breeds. A nine-point scale of the BCS was used to assess underweight (1–4 points), normal weight (5 points), and overweight (6–9 points) following Teng et al. [44]. The BCS was rated by two independent researchers by palpation of subcutaneous fat, visual assessment of the bone location and shape, and the waist of each cat. Then, the result was presented as a mean value from two measurements.

An orthopedic evaluation of the pelvic limbs was performed following Lascelles et al. [45]. The orthopedic evaluation consisted of observation and careful palpation of both knee joints, with each cat being assessed by the same experienced observer (J.B.). The observation was performed with the cat freely moving around the examination room. The palpation was performed with the cat in lateral recumbency, using minimal restraint provided by a single assistant (P.Z.). The same order was followed in every cat for the evaluation (passive observation, active observation, palpation). During the orthopedic evaluation, the lack (0) or presence (1) of local joint pain on palpation, joint swelling, joint deformities, and impaired function of the affected joint manifested by lameness was assessed. The joint pain was detected manually by palpation and considered present when withdrawal from manipulation, resists, body tenses, vocalization/increase in vocalization, orientation to the site, hissing, biting, escaping/preventing manipulation, and/or marked guarding of the palpated area were noted. The joint swelling was detected manually by palpation and considered present when an abnormal enlargement of a knee joint, typical for the accumulation of fluid, was noted. The joint deformities were detected manually by palpation and considered present when the alteration of the physiological bony shape of a knee joint was noted. The lameness was detected by passive observation and considered present when the gait or stance of a cat was abnormal. The result of the observation was confronted with the medical history data provided by the owner.

Initial inclusion criteria were based on a documented history consistent with OA and the presence of at least one clinical symptom of OA. Exclusion criteria were based on the history and radiographic signs of knee joint neoplasia, acute trauma, and/or luxation.

2.3. Radiological Data Collection

For each cat, the mediolateral projection for both knee joints was achieved. Following Lascelles et al. [9] radiographs were centered on the midpoint of the knee joint. A focus-table distance of 90 cm was used, with an exposure of 50 kVp and 2.5–3.2 mAs for the mediolateral view of the knee joints. Radiography continued until good-quality projection of the knee joint was obtained. Quality control was performed by the experienced observer (J.B.). Radiographs were taken using an X-ray system CPI Indico IQ (Communications & Power Industries Canada Inc., Georgetown, Canada). The radiographs were acquired on the computer in DICOM format using Ubuntu software (Canonical Ltd. Ubuntu Foundation, Isle of Man, Great Britain) and assessed using an advanced DICOM viewer Ginkgo CADx (GNU Lesser General Public License). The radiographic examination and image evaluation followed the international guidelines for small animal diagnostic imaging [46–48].

2.4. Data Processing

The severity of radiographic signs of knee joint OA was assessed using a scale (0–4) proposed by Lascelles et al. [9] for feline OA scoring expended by the details proposed by Kellgren and Lawrence [49] for the human knee joint OA scoring. Within the radiographic signs, the width and shape of the joint space, cortical bone surface with the presence of osteophytes and/or enthesiophytes, subchondral bone pattern with the presence of subchondral bone cyst and/sclerosis, periosteal proliferation, and intra-articular mineralization were scored as summarized in Table 1. The exemplary radiographs of scores 0–4 are presented in Figure 1.

Table 1. Radiographic signs used for scoring the severity of knee joint osteoarthritis (OA).

Score	Severity	Radiographic Signs
0	normal	normal width and shape of the joint space; smooth cortical bone surface; normal subchondral bone pattern; no periosteal proliferation; no intra-articular mineralization
1	minor	normal width and normal or irregular joint space; normal or irregular cortical bone surface; smooth subchondral bone pattern; flat periosteal proliferation; minor intra-articular mineralization
2	mild	narrow and irregular joint space with osteophytes; irregular cortical bone surface with well-defined protuberance; smooth subchondral bone pattern; flat periosteal proliferation; mild intra-articular mineralization
3	moderate	narrow and irregular joint space with multiple osteophytes, enthesiophytes, and marked asymmetry; irregular cortical bone surface with well-defined bone proliferation; subchondral bone cyst; flat periosteal proliferation; moderate intra-articular mineralization
4	severe	completely narrow joint space with large osteophytes and enthesiophytes; severe deformation of cortical bone surface; subchondral bone sclerosis; flat or intense periosteal proliferation; severe intra-articular mineralization

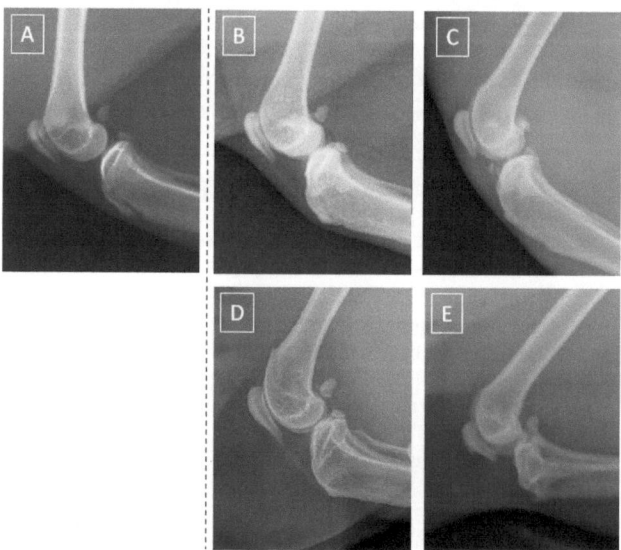

Figure 1. Exemplary mediolateral view radiographs of feline knee joints scored as normal (**A**), minor OA (**B**), mild OA (**C**), moderate OA (**D**), and severe OA (**E**). The dashed line separates the image of a normal cat knee from the images of OA knees.

2.5. Statistical Analyses

For all the statistical analyses performed, the level of significance was set at $p < 0.05$, and GraphPad Prism6 software was used (GraphPad Software Inc., San Diego, CA, USA).

2.5.1. Descriptive Statistics

For statistical analysis, the data were divided into groups regarding cats' sex, neutering, breed, and age. Each cat was also assessed using BCS in a different group as follows the underweight (UW), normal-weight (NW), or overweight (OW) group. To describe the sex, neutering, and breed groups, a total number of cats was used. For describing the age characteristics of the studied group, the minimum and maximum values, as well as $mean \pm SD$ were used. The sex structure of studied groups was compared between the UW, NW, and OW groups, and total group separately using the chi-square test. Percentage entering values were used for this test due to different group sizes. The overall severity of knee joint OA and the age structure of the studied groups were tested for normality using the Shapiro–Wilk test for each group separately. At least one data series was not normally distributed; thus, the age values and sex type occurrence were presented using the median and interquartile range, and compared between groups using the Kruskal–Wallis test. When a significant difference was evidenced, the post hoc Dunn's multiple comparisons test was used.

2.5.2. Prevalence of Symptoms and Signs of Knee Joint OA

The occurrence of each clinical symptom was annotated as 0 when not present and as 1 when present. The severity of knee joint OA was annotated as shown in Table 1. The prevalence of clinical symptoms and radiographic signs of knee joint OA was calculated for the UW, NW, OW, and total groups, separately. For comparison between the UW, NW, OW, and total groups, the chi-square test with the percentage entering values due to different group sizes was used. The occurrence of each symptom or sign was compared between groups using the Kruskal–Wallis test. When a significant difference was evidenced, the post hoc Dunn's multiple comparisons test was used. The prevalence was presented using the number of cats and the percentage (%) of each symptom or sign in each group, separately.

3. Results

3.1. Descriptive Statistics Results

Cats with a recent history of knee joint neoplasia ($n = 41$), acute trauma ($n = 14$), and/or luxation ($n = 14$) were excluded from the study. Cats with no radiographic signs of knee joint OA ($n = 536$) were excluded from the study. Finally, sixty-four ($n = 64$) cats with confirmed OA were enrolled in the study. The studied cats' group included 39 females and 25 males, aged between 1 and 20 years ($mean \pm SD$: 11.2 ± 4.8). Within those subgroups, 16 females and 13 males were neutered. Cats represented different breeds, namely 30 European Domestic Shorthair cats, 7 British Shorthair cats, 5 Devon Rex cats, 5 Maine Coon cats, 4 Ragdoll cats, 3 Bengal cats, 2 Abyssinian cats, 2 Nebelung cats, 2 Scottish Fold cats, 1 American Curl cat, 1 Cornish Rex cat, 1 Persian cat, and 1 Siberian cat. All of these cats presented radiographic signs of OA.

The UW group included 8 females and 3 males, aged between 10 and 17 years ($mean \pm SD$: 14.1 ± 2.5). Within those subgroups, 2 females and 1 male were neutered. All cats represented the European Domestic Shorthair breed. The NW group included 20 females and 15 males, aged between 1 and 20 years ($mean \pm SD$: 11.1 ± 5.2). Within those subgroups, 5 females and 6 males were neutered. These cats represented different breeds, namely 16 European Domestic Shorthair cats, 7 British Shorthair cats, 5 Devon Rex cats, 3 Bengal cats, 2 Abyssinian cats, 1 American Curl cat, and 1 Cornish Rex cat. The OW group included 11 females and 8 males, aged between 4 and 20 years ($mean \pm SD$: 9.9 ± 4.5). Within those subgroups, 9 females and 8 males were neutered. These cats represented different breeds, namely 5 Maine Coon cats, 4 Ragdoll cats, 4 European Domestic Shorthair cats, 2 Nebelung cats, 2 Scottish Fold cats, 1 Persian cat, and 1 Siberian cat.

The overall severity of knee joint osteoarthritis (OA) did not differ between the UW, NW, and OW groups ($p = 0.19$) (Figure 2A). Similarly, the age of examined cats did not differ between the UW, NW, and OW groups ($p = 0.07$) (Figure 2B). The sex structure of examined cats differed between groups as shown in Table 2. The sex structure of the OW group differed with the UW ($p < 0.0001$), NW ($p < 0.0001$), and total groups ($p < 0.0001$), respectively. However, no differences were found between the UW and NW groups ($p = 0.53$), UW and total groups ($p = 0.45$), as well as the NW and total groups ($p = 0.38$). In the OW group, the occurrence of females was lower ($p = 0.01$) (Figure 2C), and the occurrence of neutered females was higher ($p = 0.03$) (Figure 2D) than in the UW and NW groups. No differences in the occurrence of males ($p = 0.30$) (Figure 2E) and neutered males ($p = 0.30$) (Figure 2F) were noted between the studied groups.

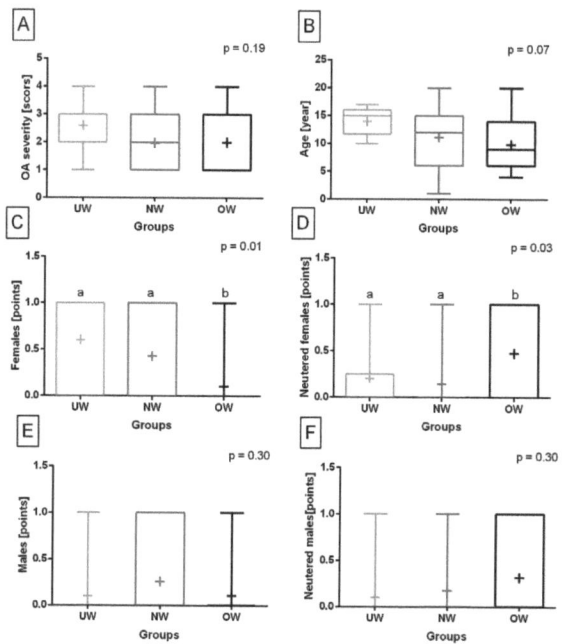

Figure 2. The overall severity of knee joint osteoarthritis (OA) (**A**), age (**B**), as well as the occurrence of females (**C**), neutered females (**D**), males (**E**), and neutered males (**F**) in the underweight (UW), normal-weight (NW), and overweight (OW) groups. Data in box plots are represented by the lower quartile, median, and upper quartile, whereas whiskers represent minimum and maximum values. Additionally, the mean values are marked by "+". Lowercase letters indicate differences between groups for $p < 0.05$.

Table 2. The sex structure of underweight (UW), normal-weight (NW), overweight (OW), and total groups. Data are represented as the number and (%) of cats representing each considered sex/neutered sex. Differences between groups are considered significant for $p < 0.05$.

Variables	UW	NW	OW	Total
Number of cats	10	35	19	64
Females	6 (60%)	15 (43%)	2 (11%)	23 (36%)
Neutered females	2 (20%)	5 (14%)	9 (47%)	16 (25%)
Males	1 (10%)	9 (26%)	2 (11%)	12 (19%)
Neutered males	1 (10%)	6 (17%)	6 (32%)	13 (20%)
Chi-square test UW NW OW		$p = 0.53$	$p < 0.0001$ $p < 0.0001$	$p = 0.45$ $p = 0.38$ $p < 0.0001$

3.2. Prevalence of Symptoms and Signs of Knee Joint OA

The prevalence of the clinical symptoms of knee joint OA differed between groups as shown in Table 3. The prevalence of the clinical symptoms in the UW group differed from the NW ($p = 0.0004$), total ($p = 0.0002$), and OW ($p = 0.0005$) groups, respectively. The prevalence of the clinical symptoms in the NW group differed with total ($p < 0.0001$) and OW ($p < 0.0001$) groups, respectively. The prevalence of the clinical symptoms in the total group also differed from the OW group ($p < 0.0001$).

Table 3. Prevalence of the clinical symptoms of knee joint osteoarthritis (OA) in underweight (UW), normal-weight (NW), overweight (OW), and total groups. Data are represented as the number and (%) of cats representing each symptom. For the sum of clinical symptoms, the medians and (interquartile ranges) are presented. Differences between groups are considered significant for $p < 0.05$.

Variables	UW	NW	OW	Total
Number of cats	10	35	19	64
Clinical symptoms				
Joint pain	2 (20%)	11 (31%)	4 (21%)	17 (27%)
Joint swelling	0 (0%)	3 (9%)	0 (0%)	3 (5%)
Joint deformities	3 (30%)	8 (23%)	4 (21%)	15 (23%)
Lameness	2 (20%)	19 (54%)	5 (26%)	26 (41%)
Reluctance to move	3 (30%)	3 (9%)	4 (21%)	10 (16%)
Apathy	9 (90%)	17 (49%)	17 (89%)	43 (67%)
Sum	2.5 (2; 4)	2 (1; 3)	2 (1; 3)	2 (1; 3)
Chi-square test				
UW		$p = 0.0004$	$p = 0.0002$	$p = 0.0005$
NW			$p < 0.0001$	$p < 0.0001$
OW				$p < 0.0001$

Concerning the consecutive clinical symptoms of knee joint OA, one may observe that joint swelling was not observed in the UW and OW groups. Among other clinical symptoms of knee joint OA, only the occurrence of apathy was higher in the NW group than in the UW and OW groups ($p = 0.003$) (Figure 3F). No differences between studied groups were found for joint pain ($p = 0.63$) (Figure 3A), joint deformities ($p = 0.86$) (Figure 3B), joint deformities ($p = 0.05$) (Figure 3C), reluctance to move ($p = 0.20$) (Figure 3D), and sum of clinical symptoms ($p = 0.41$) (Figure 3F).

The prevalence of the radiographic signs of knee joint OA differed between groups as shown in Table 4. The prevalence of the radiographic signs in the UW group differed with the OW group ($p = 0.01$) but not with the NW ($p = 0.06$) and total ($p = 0.60$). No other differences in the prevalence of the radiographic signs were found. However, concerning the consecutive radiographic signs of knee joint OA, one may observe that no differences were found in the occurrence of minor OA ($p = 0.06$ (Figure 4A), mild OA ($p = 0.42$) (Figure 4B), moderate OA ($p = 0.19$) (Figure 4C), and severe OA ($p = 0.87$) (Figure 4D) between the studied groups.

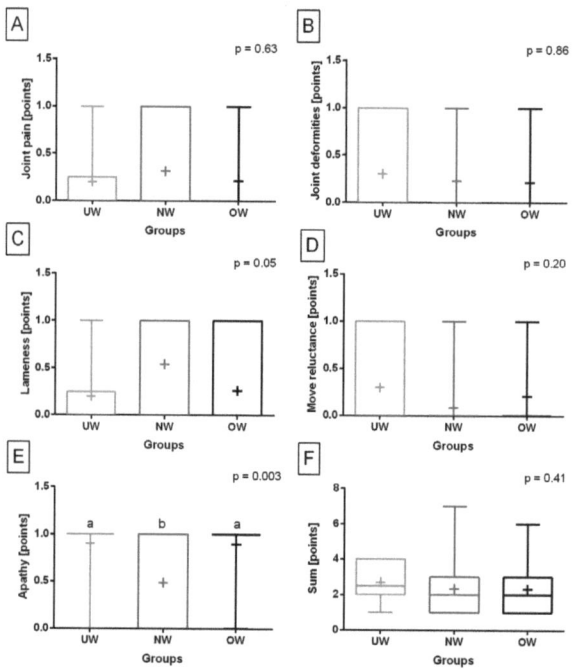

Figure 3. Occurrence of joint pain (**A**), joint deformities (**B**), lameness (**C**), reluctance to move (**D**), and apathy (**E**), as well as the sum of clinical symptoms (**F**) of knee joint osteoarthritis (OA) in the underweight (UW), normal-weight (NW), and overweight (OW) groups. Data in box plots are represented by the lower quartile, median, and upper quartile, whereas whiskers represent minimum and maximum values. Additionally, the mean values are marked by "+". Lowercase letters indicate differences between groups for $p < 0.05$.

Table 4. Prevalence of the radiographic signs of knee joint osteoarthritis (OA) all in underweight (UW), normal-weight (NW), overweight (OW), and total groups. Data are represented as the number and (%) of cats representing each sign. Differences between groups are considered significant for $p < 0.05$.

Variables	UW	NW	OW	Total
Number of cats	10	35	19	64
Radiographic signs				
Minor OA (score 1)	1 (10%)	17 (49%)	10 (53%)	28 (44%)
Mild OA (score 2)	3 (30%)	6 (17%)	2 (11%)	11 (17%)
Moderate OA (score 3)	5 (50%)	8 (23%)	4 (21%)	17 (27%)
Severe OA (score 4)	1 (10%)	4 (11%)	3 (16%)	8 (13%)
Chi-square test				
UW		$p = 0.06$	$p = 0.01$	$p = 0.13$
NW			$p = 0.60$	$p = 0.46$
OW				$p = 0.76$

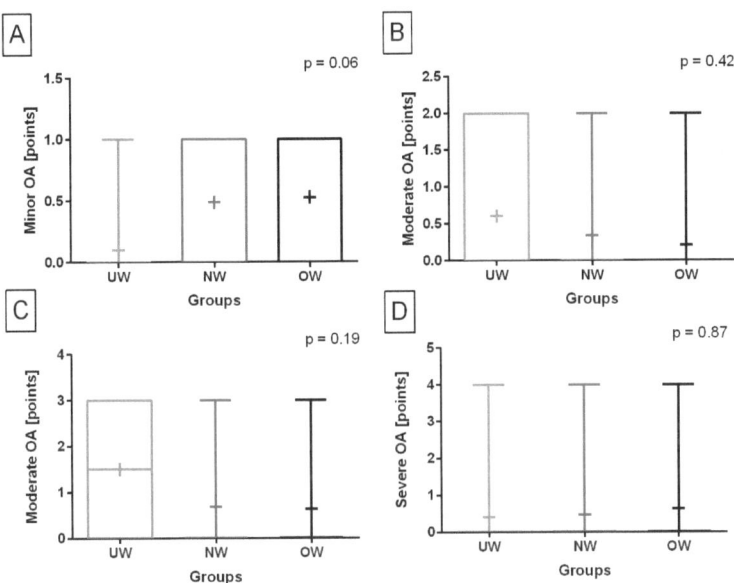

Figure 4. Occurrence of minor (**A**), mild (**B**), moderate (**C**), and severe (**D**) radiographic signs of knee joint osteoarthritis (OA) in the underweight, normal-weight, and overweight groups. Data in box plots are represented by the lower quartile, median, and upper quartile, whereas whiskers represent minimum and maximum values. Additionally, the mean values are marked by "+".

4. Discussion

To highlight the most relevant results of the current study, one may observe that the overall severity of knee joint OA did not differ between body-weight-related groups of cats. It is worth noting that the previous studies [9,45] have not compared the prevalence of the clinical symptoms and radiographic signs of feline knee joint OA depending on body weight; thus, such results are presented in the current study for the first time. Although the prevalence of the clinical symptoms and radiographic signs was different in the OW group than in other groups, the specific symptom-related difference remains unidentified. Thus, the hypothesis of the more frequent occurrence of severe knee joint OA in overweight cats can be rejected. The current study fills the gap in the research on feline knee joint OA. Lascelles et al. [9] found a very high prevalence of appendicular and axial skeleton OA in cats, and ever since OA has been considered the most common orthopedic disease of domesticated cats. Previous studies suggested the elbow [5,6,50,51] and hip [4,9,18,25] joints are the feline joints most commonly affected by OA. However, Lascelles et al. [9] reported that in the domesticated cat population, the most frequently affected joints are the hip, followed by the knee, tarsus, and then elbow [9]. Despite this important observation, studies on feline knee joint OA are scarce.

Lascelles et al. [9] evaluated the prevalence of radiographic signs of OA for the association with patient demographics, including age, body weight, sex, BCS, % time spent indoors/outdoors, vaccination status, and diet. Lascelles et al. [9] considered age to be the most essential variable that affected OA prevalence in cats, so, after accounting for age, body weight and BCS were found to not be significantly related to OA. In the Lascelles et al. [9] study, mean body weight was 5.1 ± 1.6 (range, 2.1–10.3 kg), and median BCS was 3 (range, 1–5). In the later study, Lascelles et al. [45] evaluated the relationship between radiographic signs of feline OA, clinical symptoms, and joint goniometry. Within demographic data, age, weight, BCS, and sex were considered. In the Lascelles et al. [45] study, mean body weight was 5.1 ± 1.6 (range, 2.1–10.2 kg), and median BCS was 3 (range, 1–5); thus, in [9,45], the same group of 100 cats was studied. Lascelles et al. [45] confirmed age as the most essential variable that affected the relationship between the occurrence of OA and clinical symptoms, so body weight and BCS did not change the significance of the relationship between the clinical symptoms and OA. In the current study, the overall OA severity was similar in underweight, normal-weight, and overweight cats; thus, those results are consistent with the previous studies on cats [9,45]. On the other hand, in dogs, a link between overweight and OA has been evidenced [52]. Similarly, in humans, overweight is considered to be a risk factor for the development and progression of knee joint OA; thus, weight loss is advised as the first line of the OA treatment strategy both in dogs [53] and humans [54–56]. In a case of steady weight accumulation, the opportunity to improve OA outcomes is missed [57]. One may conclude that in cats, the OA treatment strategy should consider pharmacological symptom-reducing therapy, joint supplementation, and rehabilitation [9,28,38,39], regardless of the cat's body weight.

One may state that in the studied group, overweight occurs more frequently in neutered females. This result is consistent with the previous study showing the association between cats' overweight, breed, sex, age, and neutering status [58]. However, in previous studies, contradictory to the current one, the male sex was associated with an increased risk of being overweight [58,59]. Instead, all the studies agree that neutered cats are predisposed to being overweight due to an increase in daily food intake, decrease in metabolic rate, and decrease in activity [58–60]. However, the increased risk of OA in neutered cats has not been evidenced yet, unlike neutered dogs where the OA-neutering status relationship was confirmed, but the underlying mechanism is still not fully understood [61]. Öhlund et al. [58] reported a decreased risk of being overweight in Birman and Persian breeds; however, the authors did not identify any particular cat breed at an increased risk of being overweight. In the current study, in the OW group, the Maine coon and Ragdoll cats prevailed, and all Nebelung, Scottish Fold, Persian, and Siberian cats were included. The NW group contained mostly a prevalence European Domestic Shorthair cats as well as all British Shorthair, Devon Rex, Bengal, Abyssinian, American Curl, and Cornish Rex cats.

On the other hand, in the UW group, only European Domestic Shorthair cats were included. This last observation is contradictory to the previous studies, as when comparing purebred and European Domestic Shorthair cats, the European cats were more often overweight [58,62]. To summarize breed-related factors, one may say that cat breeds can not be advised as a risk factor for being overweight [59] since no genetic factors predisposing particular cat breeds to overweight have been proven [63], whereas dog breeds, such as Golden Retriever, Pug, Beagle, English Springer Spaniel, and Border Terrier, have been proven to be predisposed to overweight [64]. It is worth noting that among considered demographic factors, age is so far the only identified risk factor affecting both prevalences of OA [8,9] and worsening of clinical symptoms of OA [45]. However, old-aged cats are less predisposed to being overweight compared with middle-aged cats [58,59,62]. The highest likelihood of being overweight was exhibited for the middle-aged cats (5 to 11 years old) [59,65] and middle-aged dogs (3 to 11 years old) [64], which are at lower risk of OA [9,52]. However, in the current study, no differences were found in the age of the cats between the body-weight-related groups. Thus, the age-related impact on the severity of knee joint OA is difficult to assess and discuss.

Scarlett and Donoghue [66] showed that overweight cats were 2.9 times as likely to be taken to veterinarians because of lameness than normal-weight cats. However, the authors just presumed that the evidenced lameness was related to OA and soft-tissue injuries. Later studies did not confirm the relationship between clinical symptoms and radiographic signs of OA and overweight [45], while the relationship between clinical symptoms and radiographic signs of OA was described in detail. Therefore, the lack of differences in lameness between the UW, NW, and OW groups evidenced in the current study may be considered consistent with the recent Lascelles et al. [45] study. Lascelles et al. [45] showed the elbow and hip joints affected by OA are most frequently found to be painful, followed by the knee and tarsus joints. The authors found joint pain in between 21% and 22% of OA-affected knee joints. Similarly, in the current study, joint pain appeared in 20%, 31%, and 21% of OA-affected knee joints in the UW, NW, and OW groups, respectively. Moreover, no differences were found between these groups. Lascelles et al. [45] also observed that the elbow joint affected by OA is most frequently found to show crepitus, effusion, and thickening followed by the knee and tarsus joints. The authors evidenced crepitus in between 10% and 14% of OA-affected knee joints, effusion in between 12% and 13% of OA-affected knee joints, and thickening in between 14% and 17% of OA-affected knee joints. As crepitus was not investigated in the current study, the appearance of joint deformities but not joint swelling ranged from 21% to 30%, with no differences between studied groups. One may note that in the current study, no joint swelling was observed in the UW or OW groups. Lascelles et al. [45] showed that the range of motion is significantly decreased in knee joints affected by OA. However, the authors reported the values of the studied range rather than the percentage of joints with a lower range of motion. In the current study, the motion decrease in OA-affected knee joints was not assessed. Lascelles et al. [45] suggested that the absence of clinical symptoms, such as pain, crepitus, effusion, and thickening of the affected joint, could be used to rule out OA. However, in the recent study, the authors did not consider non-specific symptoms, such as apathy, which seems to be the most common clinical symptom. Therefore, one may conclude that when the owner reports any unusual behavior of the cat, the veterinarian should take a detailed history driven to identify non-specific clinical symptoms of OA, especially as dogs suffering from knee joint OA most frequently show discomfort followed by other more specific clinical symptoms such as pain, limited joint range of motion, loss of muscle mass, reduced activity level, and lameness [53,67,68]. Similarly, in humans suffering from knee joint OA, joint pain and tenderness, short-term morning stiffness, and restricted movement may occur early in the disease. Crepitations, bone enlargement, and decreased range of motion suggest mild to moderate OA, whereas severe OA is characterized by pain, muscle wasting, and deformities [69].

As the future directions in the prevention of feline OA, the detailed evaluation of any behavioral changes, clinical symptoms, and cats' housing conditions should be considered. One can not rule out stress as a factor initiating the onset of OA changes in joints in cats [70–72]. Thus, further research should include the assessment of stress indicators or the collection of data on stress behaviors in history. The imaging diagnostics of feline knee joint OA should be extended by using more accurate modalities such as computed tomography [51,73] and magnetic resonance imaging [74], as it is in humans [75,76] and dogs [77]. Although conventional radiography is still the first-choice imaging modality in the diagnosis and follow-up of feline OA [9,78], its significant drawbacks such as low sensitivity and poor correlation with clinical status support the dissemination of CT- and MRI-based OA diagnosis [79].

5. Conclusions

Severe feline knee joint OA appears with similar frequency in overweight, underweight, and normal-weight cats. However, the prevalence of clinical symptoms and radiographic signs is different in overweight cats, which affects neutered females more often. Concerning consecutive symptoms and signs, it can not be unequivocally stated that the course of the disease in overweight cats is more severe. Therefore, regardless of the cat's body weight, when the owner reports any unusual behavior of the cat or changes in its behavior, the veterinarian should take a detailed history to identify non-specific clinical symptoms of OA. Thus, the veterinarian may decide to perform a radiographic examination to identify radiographic signs of OA, knowing that non-specific symptomatic cats require constant radiological monitoring to diagnose OA as early as possible and to initiate symptomatic treatment to improve their quality of life.

Author Contributions: Conceptualization, J.B.; methodology, J.B. and M.D.; software, J.B. and M.D.; validation, J.B. and M.S.; formal analysis, J.B. and M.D.; investigation, J.B., M.S. and P.Z.; resources, J.B. and P.Z.; data curation, J.B.; writing—original draft preparation, J.B., M.S. and M.D.; writing—review and editing, J.B., M.S., P.Z. and M.D.; visualization, J.B. and M.D.; supervision, M.D.; project administration, J.B. All authors have read and agreed to the published version of the manuscript.

Funding: This research received no external funding.

Institutional Review Board Statement: This research, using the results of veterinary clinical examinations, does not fall under the legislation for the protection of animals used for scientific purposes, national decree-law Dz. U. 2015 poz. 266 and 2010-63-EU directive. No ethical approval was needed.

Informed Consent Statement: Not applicable.

Data Availability Statement: The data presented in this study are available on request from the corresponding author.

Conflicts of Interest: The authors declare no conflict of interest.

References

1. Kraus, V.B.; Blanco, F.J.; Englund, M.; Karsdal, M.A.; Lohmander, L.S. Call for standardized definitions of osteoarthritis and risk stratification for clinical trials and clinical use. *Osteoarthr. Cartil.* **2015**, *23*, 1233–1241. [CrossRef] [PubMed]
2. Cope, P.; Ourradi, K.; Li, Y.; Sharif, M. Models of osteoarthritis: The good, the bad and the promising. *Osteoarthr. Cartil.* **2019**, *27*, 230–239. [CrossRef] [PubMed]
3. Nganvongpanit, K.; Soponteerakul, R.; Kaewkumpai, P.; Punyapornwithaya, V.; Buddhachat, K.; Nomsiri, R.; Kaewmong, P.; Kittiwatanawong, K.; Chawangwongsanukun, R.; Angkawanish, T.; et al. Osteoarthritis in two marine mammals and 22 land mammals: Learning from skeletal remains. *J. Anat.* **2017**, *231*, 140–155. [CrossRef] [PubMed]
4. Clarke, S.; Mellor, D.; Clements, D.; Gemmill, T.; Farrell, M.; Carmichael, S.; Bennett, D. Prevalence of radiographic signs of degenerative joint disease in a hospital population of cats. *Vet. Rec.* **2005**, *157*, 793–799. [CrossRef] [PubMed]
5. Godfrey, D. Osteoarthritis in cats: A retrospective radiological study. *J. Small Anim. Pract.* **2005**, *46*, 425–429. [CrossRef]
6. Hardie, E.M.; Roe, S.C.; Martin, F.R. Radiographic evidence of degenerative joint disease in geriatric cats: 100 cases (1994–1997). *J. Am. Vet. Med. Assoc.* **2002**, *220*, 628–632. [CrossRef]
7. Freire, M.; Robertson, I.; Bondell, H.D.; Brown, J.; Hash, J.; Pease, A.P.; Lascelles, B.D.X. Radiographic evaluation of feline appendicular degenerative joint disease vs. macroscopic appearance of articular cartilage. *Vet. Radiol. Ultrasound* **2011**, *52*, 239–247. [CrossRef]
8. Slingerland, L.; Hazewinkel, H.; Meij, B.; Picavet, P.; Voorhout, G. Cross-sectional study of the prevalence and clinical features of osteoarthritis in 100 cats. *Vet. J.* **2011**, *187*, 304–309. [CrossRef]
9. Lascelles, B.D.X.; Henry III, J.B.; Brown, J.; Robertson, I.; Sumrell, A.T.; Simpson, W.; Wheeler, S.; Hansen, B.D.; Zamprogno, H.; Freire, M.; et al. Cross-sectional study of the prevalence of radiographic degenerative joint disease in domesticated cats. *Vet. Surg.* **2010**, *39*, 535–544. [CrossRef]
10. Gandolfi, B.; Alamri, S.; Darby, W.; Adhikari, B.; Lattimer, J.; Malik, R.; Wade, C.M.; Lyons, L.A.; Cheng, J.; Bateman, J.F.; et al. A dominant TRPV4 variant underlies osteochondrodysplasia in Scottish fold cats. *Osteoarthr. Cartil.* **2016**, *24*, 1441–1450. [CrossRef]
11. Macri, B.; Marino, F.; Mazzullo, G.; Trusso, A.; De Maria, R.; Amedeo, S.; Divari, S.; Castagnaro, M. Mucopolysaccharidosis VI in a Siamese/short-haired European cat. *J. Vet. Med. Ser. A* **2002**, *49*, 438–442. [CrossRef]
12. Valastro, C.; Di Bello, A.; Crovace, A. Congenital elbow subluxation in a cat. *Vet. Radiol. Ultrasound* **2005**, *46*, 63–64. [CrossRef]
13. Lemetayer, J.; Taylor, S. Inflammatory joint disease in cats: Diagnostic approach and treatment. *J. Feline Med. Surg.* **2014**, *16*, 547–562. [CrossRef]
14. Keller, G.; Reed, A.; Lattimer, J.; Corley, E. Hip dysplasia: A feline population study. *Vet. Radiol. Ultrasound* **1999**, *40*, 460–464. [CrossRef]
15. Perry, K. Feline hip dysplasia: A challenge to recognise and treat. *J. Feline Med. Surg.* **2016**, *18*, 203–218. [CrossRef]
16. Prior, J. Luxating patellae in Devon rex cats. *Vet. Rec.* **1985**, *117*, 154–155. [CrossRef]
17. Hamish, R.D.; Butterworth, S. *A Guide to Canine and Feline Orthopaedic Surgery*; Blackwell Science Ltd, Cap: Oxford, UK, 2000; Volume 12, p. 91.
18. Černá, P.; Timmermans, J.; Komenda, D.; Nývltová, I.; Proks, P. The Prevalence of Feline Hip Dysplasia, Patellar Luxation and Lumbosacral Transitional Vertebrae in Pedigree Cats in The Czech Republic. *Animals* **2021**, *11*, 2482. [CrossRef]
19. Houlton, J.; Meynink, S. Medial patellar luxation in the cat. *J. Small Anim. Pract.* **1989**, *30*, 349–352. [CrossRef]
20. Woodell-May, J.E.; Sommerfeld, S.D. Role of inflammation and the immune system in the progression of osteoarthritis. *J. Orthop. Res.* **2020**, *38*, 253–257. [CrossRef]
21. Hunter, D.J. Pharmacologic therapy for osteoarthritis—the era of disease modification. *Nat. Rev. Rheumatol.* **2011**, *7*, 13–22. [CrossRef]

22. Ramírez-Flores, G.I.; Del Angel-Caraza, J.; Quijano-Hernández, I.A.; Hulse, D.A.; Beale, B.S.; Victoria-Mora, J.M. Correlation between osteoarthritic changes in the stifle joint in dogs and the results of orthopedic, radiographic, ultrasonographic and arthroscopic examinations. *Vet. Res. Commun.* **2017**, *41*, 129–137. [CrossRef] [PubMed]
23. Klinck, M.P.; Frank, D.; Guillot, M.; Troncy, E. Owner-perceived signs and veterinary diagnosis in 50 cases of feline osteoarthritis. *Can. Vet. J.* **2012**, *53*, 1181.
24. Klinck, M.P.; Rialland, P.; Guillot, M.; Moreau, M.; Frank, D.; Troncy, E. Preliminary validation and reliability testing of the Montreal Instrument for Cat Arthritis Testing, for use by veterinarians, in a colony of laboratory cats. *Animals* **2015**, *5*, 1252–1267. [CrossRef]
25. Lascelles, B.D.X.; Hansen, B.D.; Roe, S.; DePuy, V.; Thomson, A.; Pierce, C.C.; Smith, E.S.; Rowinski, E. Evaluation of client-specific outcome measures and activity monitoring to measure pain relief in cats with osteoarthritis. *J. Vet. Intern. Med.* **2007**, *21*, 410–416. [CrossRef] [PubMed]
26. Bennett, D.; Zainal Ariffin, S.M.b.; Johnston, P. Osteoarthritis in the cat: 1. How common is it and how easy to recognise? *J. Feline Med. Surg.* **2012**, *14*, 65–75. [CrossRef] [PubMed]
27. Godfrey, D.; Vaughan, L. Historical prevalence of radiological appendicular osteoarthritis in cats (1972–1973). *J. Am. Anim. Hosp. Assoc.* **2018**, *54*, 209–212. [CrossRef]
28. Bennett, D.; Morton, C. A study of owner observed behavioural and lifestyle changes in cats with musculoskeletal disease before and after analgesic therapy. *J. Feline Med. Surg.* **2009**, *11*, 997–1004. [CrossRef]
29. KuKanich, K.; George, C.; Roush, J.K.; Sharp, S.; Farace, G.; Yerramilli, M.; Peterson, S.; Grauer, G.F. Effects of low-dose meloxicam in cats with chronic kidney disease. *J. Feline Med. Surg.* **2021**, *23*, 138–148. [CrossRef]
30. Gunew, M.N.; Menrath, V.H.; Marshall, R.D. Long-term safety, efficacy and palatability of oral meloxicam at 0.01–0.03 mg/kg for treatment of osteoarthritic pain in cats. *J. Feline Med. Surg.* **2008**, *10*, 235–241. [CrossRef]
31. King, J.N.; King, S.; Budsberg, S.C.; Lascelles, B.D.X.; Bienhoff, S.E.; Roycroft, L.M.; Roberts, E.S. Clinical safety of robenacoxib in feline osteoarthritis: Results of a randomized, blinded, placebo-controlled clinical trial. *J. Feline Med. Surg.* **2016**, *18*, 632–642.
32. Kongara, K.; Chambers, J.P. Robenacoxib in the treatment of pain in cats and dogs: Safety, efficacy, and place in therapy. *Vet. Med. Res. Rep.* **2018**, *9*, 53–61.
33. Guedes, V.; Castro, J.P.; Brito, I. Topical capsaicin for pain in osteoarthritis: A literature review. *Reumatol. Clín. Engl. Ed.* **2018**, *14*, 40–45. [CrossRef]
34. Guedes, A.G.; Meadows, J.M.; Pypendop, B.H.; Johnson, E.G.; Zaffarano, B. Assessment of the effects of gabapentin on activity levels and owner-perceived mobility impairment and quality of life in osteoarthritic geriatric cats. *J. Am. Vet. Med. Assoc.* **2018**, *253*, 579–585. [CrossRef]
35. Gruen, M.E.; Myers, J.A.; Lascelles, B.D.X. Efficacy and safety of an anti-nerve growth factor antibody (frunevetmab) for the treatment of degenerative joint disease-associated chronic pain in cats: A multisite pilot field study. *Front. Vet. Sci.* **2021**, *8*, 610028.
36. Gruen, M.E.; Myers, J.A.; Tena, J.K.S.; Becskei, C.; Cleaver, D.M.; Lascelles, B.D.X. Frunevetmab, a felinized anti-nerve growth factor monoclonal antibody, for the treatment of pain from osteoarthritis in cats. *J. Vet. Intern. Med.* **2021**, *35*, 2752–2762. [CrossRef]
37. Bradshaw, J. Normal feline behaviour:... and why problem behaviours develop. *J. Feline Med. Surg.* **2018**, *20*, 411–421. [CrossRef]
38. Drum, M.G.; Bockstahler, B.; Levine, D.; Marcellin-Little, D.J. Feline rehabilitation. *Vet. Clin. Small Anim. Pract.* **2015**, *45*, 185–201. [CrossRef]
39. Johnson, K.A.; Lee, A.H.; Swanson, K.S. Nutrition and nutraceuticals in the changing management of osteoarthritis for dogs and cats. *J. Am. Vet. Med. Assoc.* **2020**, *256*, 1335–1341. [CrossRef]
40. Clarke, S.; Bennett, D. Feline osteoarthritis: A prospective study of 28 cases. *J. Small Anim. Pract.* **2006**, *47*, 439–445. [CrossRef]
41. Leijon, A.; Ley, C.J.; Corin, A.; Ley, C. Cartilage lesions in feline stifle joints–Associations with articular mineralizations and implications for osteoarthritis. *Res. Vet. Sci.* **2017**, *114*, 186–193. [CrossRef]
42. Voss, K.; Karli, P.; Montavon, P.M.; Geyer, H. Association of mineralisations in the stifle joint of domestic cats with degenerative joint disease and cranial cruciate ligament pathology. *J. Feline Med. Surg.* **2017**, *19*, 27–35. [CrossRef] [PubMed]
43. Freire, M.; Brown, J.; Robertson, I.D.; Pease, A.P.; Hash, J.; Hunter, S.; Simpson, W.; Thomson Sumrell, A.; Lascelles, B.D.X. Meniscal mineralization in domestic cats. *Vet. Surg.* **2010**, *39*, 545–552. [CrossRef] [PubMed]
44. Teng, K.T.; McGreevy, P.D.; Toribio, J.A.L.; Raubenheimer, D.; Kendall, K.; Dhand, N.K. Strong associations of nine-point body condition scoring with survival and lifespan in cats. *J. Feline Med. Surg.* **2018**, *20*, 1110–1118. [CrossRef] [PubMed]
45. Lascelles, B.D.X.; Dong, Y.H.; Marcellin-Little, D.J.; Thomson, A.; Wheeler, S.; Correa, M. Relationship of orthopedic examination, goniometric measurements, and radiographic signs of degenerative joint disease in cats. *BMC Vet. Res.* **2012**, *8*, 1–8. [CrossRef] [PubMed]
46. PECK, G. *Manual of Small Animal Diagnostic Imaging*; Wiley Online Library: Hoboken, NJ, USA, 1995.
47. Morgan, J.P.; Wolvekamp, P. *Atlas of Radiology of the Traumatized Dog and Cat: The Case-Based Approach*, 2nd ed.; Schlütersche: Magdeburg, Germany, 2010.
48. Kirberger, R.M.; McEvoy, F.J. *BSAVA Manual of Canine and Feline Musculoskeletal Imaging*; British Small Animal Veterinary Association: Quedgeley, UK, 2016.
49. Kellgren, J.H.; Lawrence, J. Radiological assessment of osteo-arthrosis. *Ann. Rheum. Dis.* **1957**, *16*, 494. [CrossRef] [PubMed]
50. Freire, M.; Meuten, D.; Lascelles, D. Pathology of articular cartilage and synovial membrane from elbow joints with and without degenerative joint disease in domestic cats. *Vet. Pathol.* **2014**, *51*, 968–978. [CrossRef]

51. Ley, C.J.; Leijon, A.; Uhlhorn, M.; Marcelino, L.; Hansson, K.; Ley, C. Computed tomography is superior to radiography for detection of feline elbow osteoarthritis. *Res. Vet. Sci.* **2021**, *140*, 6–17. [CrossRef]
52. Marshall, W.; Bockstahler, B.; Hulse, D.; Carmichael, S. A review of osteoarthritis and obesity: Current understanding of the relationship and benefit of obesity treatment and prevention in the dog. *Vet. Comp. Orthop. Traumatol.* **2009**, *22*, 339–345.
53. Budsberg, S.C. Medical therapy for stifle osteoarthritis. In *Advances in the Canine Cranial Cruciate Ligament*; Wiley Online Library: Hoboken, NJ, USA, 2017; pp. 333–341.
54. Bliddal, H.; Leeds, A.; Christensen, R. Osteoarthritis, obesity and weight loss: Evidence, hypotheses and horizons–a scoping review. *Obes. Rev.* **2014**, *15*, 578–586.
55. Grotle, M.; Hagen, K.B.; Natvig, B.; Dahl, F.A.; Kvien, T.K. Obesity and osteoarthritis in knee, hip and/or hand: An epidemiological study in the general population with 10 years follow-up. *BMC Musculoskelet. Disord.* **2008**, *9*, 1–5.
56. Reijman, M.; Pols, H.; Bergink, A.; Hazes, J.; Belo, J.; Lievense, A.; Bierma-Zeinstra, S. Body mass index associated with onset and progression of osteoarthritis of the knee but not of the hip: The Rotterdam Study. *Ann. Rheum. Dis.* **2007**, *66*, 158–162.
57. Lim, Y.Z.; Wong, J.; Hussain, M.; Estee, M.M.; Zolio, L.; Page, M.J.; Harrison, C.L.; Wluka, A.E.; Wang, Y.; Cicuttini, F.M. Recommendations for weight management in osteoarthritis: A systematic review of clinical practice guidelines. *Osteoarthr. Cartil. Open* **2022**, *4*, 100298.
58. Öhlund, M.; Palmgren, M.; Holst, B.S. Overweight in adult cats: A cross-sectional study. *Acta Vet. Scand.* **2018**, *60*, 1–10. [CrossRef]
59. Courcier, E.; Mellor, D.; Pendlebury, E.; Evans, C.; Yam, P. An investigation into the epidemiology of feline obesity in Great Britain: Results of a cross-sectional study of 47 companion animal practises. *Vet. Rec.* **2012**, *171*, 560. [PubMed]
60. Kanchuk, M.L.; Backus, R.C.; Calvert, C.C.; Morris, J.G.; Rogers, Q.R. Weight gain in gonadectomized normal and lipoprotein lipase–deficient male domestic cats results from increased food intake and not decreased energy expenditure. *J. Nutr.* **2003**, *133*, 1866–1874. [CrossRef] [PubMed]
61. Anderson, K.L.; O'Neill, D.G.; Brodbelt, D.C.; Church, D.B.; Meeson, R.L.; Sargan, D.; Summers, J.F.; Zulch, H.; Collins, L.M. Prevalence, duration and risk factors for appendicular osteoarthritis in a UK dog population under primary veterinary care. *Sci. Rep.* **2018**, *8*, 5641. [CrossRef] [PubMed]
62. Teng, K.T.; McGreevy, P.D.; Toribio, J.A.L.; Raubenheimer, D.; Kendall, K.; Dhand, N.K. Risk factors for underweight and overweight in cats in metropolitan Sydney, Australia. *Prev. Vet. Med.* **2017**, *144*, 102–111.
63. Tarkosova, D.; Story, M.; Rand, J.; Svoboda, M. Feline obesity–prevalence, risk factors, pathogenesis, associated conditions and assessment: A review. *Veter. Med.* **2016**, *61*, 295–307.
64. Pegram, C.; Raffan, E.; White, E.; Ashworth, A.; Brodbelt, D.; Church, D.; O'Neill, D. Frequency, breed predisposition and demographic risk factors for overweight status in dogs in the UK. *J. Small Anim. Pract.* **2021**, *62*, 521–530.
65. Colliard, L.; Paragon, B.M.; Lemuet, B.; Bénet, J.J.; Blanchard, G. Prevalence and risk factors of obesity in an urban population of healthy cats. *J. Feline Med. Surg.* **2009**, *11*, 135–140. [CrossRef]
66. Scarlett, J.; Donoghue, S. Associations between body condition and disease in cats. *J. Am. Vet. Med. Assoc.* **1998**, *212*, 1725–1731.
67. Teunissen, M.; Mastbergen, S.C.; Spoelman, D.C.; Lafeber, F.P.; Ludwig, I.S.; Broere, F.; Tryfonidou, M.A.; Meij, B.P. Knee joint distraction in a dog as treatment for severe osteoarthritis. *VCOT Open* **2022**, *5*, e11–e17. [CrossRef]
68. Lee, S.H.; Roh, Y.H.; Lee, D.B.; Cho, J.H.; Kim, C.H. Stifle Joint Arthrodesis for Treating Chronic-Osteoarthritis-Affected Dogs. *Vet. Sci.* **2023**, *10*, 407. [CrossRef]
69. Watts, R.A.; Conaghan, P.G.; Denton, C.; Foster, H.; Isaacs, J.; Müller-Ladner, U. Clinical features of osteoarthritis. In *Oxford Textbook of Rheumatology*, 4th ed.; Oxford University Press: Oxford, UK, 2013.
70. Buffington, C.T.; Bain, M. Stress and feline health. *Vet. Clin. Small Anim. Pract.* **2020**, *50*, 653–662. [CrossRef]
71. Yaribeygi, H.; Panahi, Y.; Sahraei, H.; Johnston, T.P.; Sahebkar, A. The impact of stress on body function: A review. *EXCLI J.* **2017**, *16*, 1057.
72. Stella, J.; Croney, C.; Buffington, T. Effects of stressors on the behavior and physiology of domestic cats. *Appl. Anim. Behav. Sci.* **2013**, *143*, 157–163. [CrossRef]
73. Boyd, S.; Müller, R.; Leonard, T.; Herzog, W. Long-term periarticular bone adaptation in a feline knee injury model for post-traumatic experimental osteoarthritis. *Osteoarthr. Cartil.* **2005**, *13*, 235–242. [CrossRef]
74. Del Vecchio, O.V. Magnetic resonance imaging findings in a cat with cranial cruciate ligament rupture. *Vet. Rec. Case Rep.* **2021**, *9*, e91. [CrossRef]
75. Ciliberti, F.K.; Guerrini, L.; Gunnarsson, A.E.; Recenti, M.; Jacob, D.; Cangiano, V.; Tesfahunegn, Y.A.; Islind, A.S.; Tortorella, F.; Tsirilaki, M.; et al. CT-and MRI-based 3D reconstruction of knee joint to assess cartilage and bone. *Diagnostics* **2022**, *12*, 279. [CrossRef]
76. Du, Y.; Almajalid, R.; Shan, J.; Zhang, M. A novel method to predict knee osteoarthritis progression on MRI using machine learning methods. *IEEE Trans. Nanobiosci.* **2018**, *17*, 228–236. [CrossRef]
77. Chung, C.S.; Tu, Y.J.; Lin, L.S. Comparison of Digital Radiography, Computed Tomography, and Magnetic Resonance Imaging Features in Canine Spontaneous Degenerative Stifle Joint Osteoarthritis. *Animals* **2023**, *13*, 849. [CrossRef] [PubMed]

78. Perry, K. Feline osteoarthritis: Diagnosis and management. In *BSAVA Congress Proceedings 2019*; BSAVA Library: Quedgeley, UK, 2019; pp. 404–405.
79. Steenkamp, W.; Rachuene, P.A.; Dey, R.; Mzayiya, N.L.; Ramasuvha, B.E. The correlation between clinical and radiological severity of osteoarthritis of the knee. *SICOT J.* **2022**, *8*, 14. [CrossRef] [PubMed]

Disclaimer/Publisher's Note: The statements, opinions and data contained in all publications are solely those of the individual author(s) and contributor(s) and not of MDPI and/or the editor(s). MDPI and/or the editor(s) disclaim responsibility for any injury to people or property resulting from any ideas, methods, instructions or products referred to in the content.

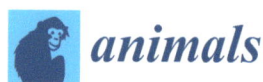

Article

A Preliminary Report on the Combined Effect of Intra-Articular Platelet-Rich Plasma Injections and Photobiomodulation in Canine Osteoarthritis

J. C. Alves [1,2,3,4,*], Ana Santos [1] and L. Miguel Carreira [5,6,7]

1. Divisão de Medicina Veterinária, Guarda Nacional Republicana (GNR), Rua Presidente Arriaga, 9, 1200-771 Lisbon, Portugal
2. Faculty of Veterinary Medicine, Lusófona University, 1749-024 Lisbon, Portugal
3. Centro de Ciência Animal e Veterinária, Lusófona University, 1749-024 Lisbon, Portugal
4. MED—Mediterranean Institute for Agriculture, Environment and Development, Instituto de Investigação e Formação Avançada, Universidade de Évora, Pólo da Mitra, Ap. 94, 7006-554 Évora, Portugal
5. Faculty of Veterinary Medicine, University of Lisbon (FMV/ULisboa), 1300-477 Lisbon, Portugal; miguelcarreira@fmv.ulisboa.pt
6. Interdisciplinary Centre for Research in Animal Health (CIISA), University of Lisbon (FMV/ULisboa), 1649-004 Lisbon, Portugal
7. Anjos of Assis Veterinary Medicine Centre (CMVAA), 2830-077 Barreiro, Portugal
* Correspondence: alves.jca@gnr.pt

Simple Summary: Osteoarthritis is a very common joint disease in dogs, and clinicians usually favor a multimodal approach for the management of the disease. There has been a growing interest concerning platelet-rich plasma and photobiomodulation, alongside an increasing body of evidence supporting their use. Although there are studies reporting the effect of these treatments individually, there is still a lack of information on their combined use. We aimed to evaluate the effect of the intra-articular administration of platelet-rich plasma, photobiomodulation, and their combined use in dogs with bilateral hip osteoarthritis. Our results show that combining the two treatments leads to greater, longer-lasting clinical improvements.

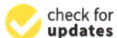

Citation: Alves, J.C.; Santos, A.; Carreira, L.M. A Preliminary Report on the Combined Effect of Intra-Articular Platelet-Rich Plasma Injections and Photobiomodulation in Canine Osteoarthritis. *Animals* 2023, 13, 3247. https://doi.org/10.3390/ani13203247

Academic Editor: Clive J. C. Phillips

Received: 7 September 2023
Revised: 13 October 2023
Accepted: 17 October 2023
Published: 18 October 2023

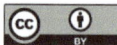

Copyright: © 2023 by the authors. Licensee MDPI, Basel, Switzerland. This article is an open access article distributed under the terms and conditions of the Creative Commons Attribution (CC BY) license (https://creativecommons.org/licenses/by/4.0/).

Abstract: Osteoarthritis (OA) is highly prevalent in the canine population. Due to the multiple dimensions of the disease, a multimodal approach is usually favored by clinicians. To evaluate the combined treatment with intra-articular platelet-rich plasma (PRP) and photobiomodulation in dogs with bilateral hip OA, thirty dogs were assigned to a PRP group (PRPG, n = 10), a photobiomodulation group (PBMTG, n = 10), or a combined therapies group (PRP+PBMTG, n = 10). The PRPG received two intra-articular administrations of platelet-rich plasma 14 days apart. The PBMTG received photobiomodulation with a therapeutic laser, with three sessions every other day in week one; two sessions in week two; a single session in week three; and one session/month on follow-up evaluation days. The PRP+PBMTG received the two combined therapies. The response to treatment was evaluated with weight-bearing distribution and the Canine Brief Pain Inventory, the Liverpool Osteoarthritis in Dogs, and the Canine Orthopedic Index. Evaluations were conducted before treatment and +8, +15, +30, +60, and +90 days after initial treatment. Normality was assessed with a Shapiro–Wilk test, and the groups' results in each evaluation moment were compared using a Mann–Whitney U test. Animals of both sexes (male n = 19, female n = 11) were included in the sample, with a mean age of 7.8 ± 2.5 years and a body weight of 26.5 ± 4.7 kg. Joints were classified as mild (n = 6, three in PRPG, two in PBMTG, and one in PRP+PBMTG), moderate (n = 18, six in PRPG, five in PBMTG, and seven in PRP+PBMTG), and severe (n = 6, one in PRPG, three in PBMTG, and two in PRP+PBMTG). No differences were found between groups at the initial evaluation. All treatments produced clinically significant improvements compared to the assessment on treatment day. The combination of PRP and photobiomodulation produced greater, longer-lasting improvements. PRP and photobiomodulation can improve objective outcomes and client-reported outcome measures in dogs with OA. Their combined use leads to greater, longer-lasting, clinically significant improvements.

Keywords: dog; osteoarthritis; chronic pain; orthopedics; platelet-rich plasma; regenerative therapy; photobiomodulation

1. Introduction

Osteoarthritis (OA) has a high prevalence in the canine population, and the disease significantly impacts the patient's overall quality of life, as it produces pain and affects joint function and mobility [1–4]. Adequate disease management is still challenging, as reflected in the broad number of therapeutic approaches described [5,6]. Due to the multiple dimensions of the disease, a multimodal approach is usually favored by clinicians [7].

Autologous platelet therapies are an interesting approach, as platelets are a part of the body's natural response to injury. Attributed effects include a reduction in inflammation and a contribution to tissue regeneration. At the joint level, platelet-rich plasma (PRP) can promote cartilage synthesis or inhibit its breakdown [8,9]. The use of PRP has been described for the treatment of different musculoskeletal conditions in dogs, such as OA, tendinopathies, or muscle injury [10,11], but the described effects vary significantly between reports. This variability is likely related to various compositions and characteristics of PRP products regarding concentration and numbers of platelet, leukocytes, and red blood cells [12,13].

Photobiomodulation therapy (PBMT) has also gained increasing interest based on the ability of red/near infrared light to produce a clinical effect, including stimulation of tissue healing, analgesia, and reduced inflammation [14]. It has been described in dogs as managing various conditions, such as OA, gingivostomatitis, wound healing, and even diarrhea [15–19]. The results obtained with PBMT in managing osteoarthritis are attributed to the effect of the delivered photons that dissociate inhibitory nitric oxide while increasing electron transport and ATP production. It also increases the expression of genes that increase protein synthesis, particularly anti-apoptotic proteins, and antioxidant enzymes, leading to cell proliferation and anti-inflammatory signaling [15]. As for PRP, a variability in described effects of PBMT is also found in the available literature, likely linked to the difference in selected parameters [17].

Having objective measures to evaluate patients and determine response to treatment is paramount. The evaluation of weight bearing, off-loading, and limb favoring are evaluations commonly performed during the orthopedic exam [20,21]. In OA cases, some patients may exhibit only discrete lameness at a walk or a trot while showing changes in weight-bearing distribution at a stance in response to pain [22,23]. In fact, stance analysis has been shown to be sensitive in identifying dog lameness [24]. In addition to objective measures, several client-reported outcome measures have been developed to assess OA patients. They can identify changes and degrees of a pet's subjective status, and owners can also interpret changes over an extended period of time [25,26]. The client-reported outcome measures aimed at dogs with OA include the Liverpool Osteoarthritis in Dogs (LOAD) [27,28], the Canine Orthopedic Index (COI) [29], and the Canine Brief Pain Inventory (CBPI) [30]. They have been recommended for use in dogs with OA in a recent COSMIN-based systemic review [31] and in WSAVA guidelines for the recognition assessment and treatment of pain [32].

This study aimed to evaluate the combined treatment with intra-articular PRP and PBMT in dogs with bilateral hip OA. It will serve as a preliminary study to determine adequate treatment parameters and frequency. We hypothesized that combining the two treatments would better alleviate OA-related clinical signs than their isolated use.

2. Materials and Methods

The study protocol was approved by the ethical review committee of the University of Évora (Órgão Responsável pelo Bem-Estar dos Animais da Universidade de Évora, approval no. GD/16901/2022). All methods were carried out in accordance with relevant guidelines and regulations, complying with ARRIVE guidelines. Informed consent and permission were obtained in writing from the institution responsible for the animals (Guarda Nacional Republicana, Portuguese Gendarmerie).

Thirty dogs with bilateral hip OA were recruited. All animals had a consistent history, with the canine handler trainer referring specific complaints, such as difficulty rising, jumping, and maintaining obedience positions. Pain during joint mobilization, stiffness, and reduced range of motion was elicited on physical examination. Radiographic findings were consistent with bilateral hip OA (Orthopedic Foundation for Animals' hip scores of mild, moderate, or severe) [33]. Animals were >2 years old, had a body weight > 20 kg, and were without any other medications or nutritional supplements administered for >6 weeks. Animals with other orthopedic, neurologic, or other diseases were excluded. Since all animals had clinical signs of OA, a placebo group was not included for ethical reasons. However, these treatments have been evaluated compared to a placebo or control before [11,16].

After selection, patients were randomly assigned a PRP group (PRPG, n = 10), a PBMT group (PBMTG, n = 10), or a combined therapies group (PRP+PBMTG, n = 10). Since all animals had bilateral hip OA, both joints of each patient received the same treatment [11,16]. The PRPG received two intra-articular administrations of 2 mL of PRP per hip joint, produced with the commercially available CRT PurePRP® Kit (Companion Regenerative Therapies, Newark, DE, USA). One was administered on day 0, and, in accordance with the manufacturer's recommendations, a follow-up administration was performed 14 days after the initial treatment. For the preparation of PRP, 50 mL of whole blood was collected from the patient's jugular vein directly into a 60 mL syringe filled with 10 mL of Anticoagulant Citrate Dextrose Solution. After collection, the blood was transferred and loaded into a concentrating device. The device was then placed in a centrifuge (Executive Series Centrifuge II, Companion Regenerative Therapies, Newark, DE, USA) and spun at 3600 rpm for 1 min. After the first centrifugation, the buffy coat and platelet-poor plasm were collected, transferred to a second concentrating device, and spun at 3800 rpm for 5 min. After the second centrifugation process, the remaining platelet-poor plasma was removed until 4 mL was left. The device was then swirled to resuspend the platelets, and the 4 mL of PRP was aspirated into a 12 mL syringe. The PRP was administered immediately after preparation, without activation.

PRP and whole blood samples were sent to an external lab for analysis. Compositions were determined and compared. The intra-articular administration was conducted under light sedation, obtained with the simultaneous intravenous administration of medetomidine (0.01 mg/kg) and butorphanol (0.1 mg/kg). The procedure for hip intra-articular administrations has been described before [6]. The animal was placed in lateral recumbency, with the joint being assessed at that moment upward. A 4 × 4 cm window, with the greater trochanter in the center, was clipped and aseptically prepared. An assistant then placed the limb in a neutral position parallel to the table. A 21-gauge with a 2.5″ length needle was then introduced just dorsal to the greater trochanter, perpendicular to the limb's long axis until the joint was reached. Correct needle placement was confirmed by collecting synovial fluid.

The PBMTG received PBMT with a therapeutic laser (CTS-DUO Class IV Laser, Companion Animal Health, Enovis, Wilmington, DE, USA). The hair was clipped (for blinding purposes), and no sedation was required for PBMT. Sessions were conducted for three consecutive weeks in the following fashion: in week one, three sessions every other day; in week two, two sessions, two days apart; in week three, a single session. After this first treatment period, a single session was conducted monthly on follow-up evaluation days. PBMT parameters are presented in Table 1 and were selected based on the manufacturer's recommendation and previous evidence of a positive therapeutic effect [16].

Animals in the PRP+PBMTG were treated with the two combined therapies on the same schedule as the PRPG and the PBMTG. All groups were prescribed a 3-day rest period following the days of the IA administrations for the PRPG and the PRP+PBMTG.

Table 1. Photobiomodulation therapy treatment parameters.

	Light Parameters (Dose)
Wavelength (nm)	980 nm
Radiant Power (W)	13
Irradiance (W/cm^2) at the skin surface	2.6 (using a large contact treatment head)
Fluence (J/cm^2)	15
Total Joules	5250
Treatment Protocol	Continuously moving grid pattern in contact over the treatment area at a speed of 2.5–7.5 cm/s, according to manufacturer recommendations.
Treatment Area (cm^2)	350 (entire hip area)
Treatment Time	6 min, 44 s

The follow-up evaluations were conducted at scheduled moments on days 14 (+14 d, before the second IA PRP administration), 30 (+30 d), and 90 (+90 d) after the initial treatment. At the follow-up moments, a weight-bearing evaluation was conducted (Companion Stance Analyser; Enovis®, Newark, DE, USA). The procedure of weight-bearing evaluation was performed as described before [34]. The equipment was placed in the center of a room, at least 1 m from the walls. After zeroing the equipment, dogs were encouraged to stand on the platform, ensuring that one foot was placed on each quadrant. At least twenty measurements were obtained for each patient, and the mean value was determined. After weight-bearing distribution values were collected, a deviation from the normal weight distribution for pelvic limbs was calculated by subtracting the weight-bearing of the limb from the considered normal of 20% [23]. In addition, a left-right symmetry index (SI) was also calculated with the formula: $SI = [(WBR - WBL)/((WBR + WBL) \times 0.5)] \times 100$, where WBR is the weight-bearing for the right limb, and WBL is the weight-bearing for the left limb [28,35]. Negative values were made positive. In addition to the weight-bearing distribution evaluation, a digital copy of the CBPI, the LOAD, and the COI were completed sequentially by the same handler, blinded to their dog's treatment group. All have previously been validated in Portuguese versions [36–39].

All of the described procedures were performed by the same researcher, who was kept blinded to the dogs' treatment group. Data were assessed with a Shapiro–Wilk test for the evaluation of normal distribution. In each evaluation moment, the groups' results were compared using a Mann–Whitney U test. All results were analyzed with IBM SPSS Statistics version 20. Statistical significance was considered at $p < 0.05$.

3. Results

Animals of both sexes were included in the present sample (18 males, eight in PRPG, five in PBMTG, and five in PRP+PBMTG; and 12 females, two in PRPG, five in PBMTG, and five in PRP+PBMTG), having a mean age of 7.8 ± 2.5 years (7.6 ± 1.9 in PRPG, 7.9 ± 2.4 in PBMTG, and 7.4 ± 2.8 in PRP+PBMTG). All had an ideal body condition score for working dogs of 4/9 (n = 24) and 5/9 (n = 6) on the Laflamme scale [40], with a mean body weight of 26.5 ± 4.7kg (26.4 ± 2.4 in PRPG, 27.3 ± 5.2 in PBMTG, and 24.9 ± 4.6 in PRP+PBMTG). Four dog breeds were present in the sample, similar to those found in most police and working dog populations throughout the world: German Shepherd Dogs (n = 11, three in PRPG, four in PBMTG, and four in PRP+PBMTG), Belgian Malinois Shepherd Dogs (n = 9, four in PRPG, two in PBMTG, and three in PRP+PBMTG), Labrador Retriever (n = 6, two in PRPG, two in PBMTG, and two in PRP+PBMTG), and Dutch Shepherd Dogs (n = 4, one in PRPG, two in PBMTG, and one in PRP+PBMTG). The dogs were used in drug detection and patrol work. Hips were graded with the OFA hip grading scheme, and six animals were classified as mild (three in PRPG, two in PBMTG, and one in PRP+PBMTG), 18 as moderate (six in PRPG, five in PBMTG, and seven in PRP+PBMTG), and six as severe (one in PRPG, three in PBMTG, and two in PRP+PBMTG). All patients were followed up to the last evaluation moment (+90 days), and during this period, no additional treatment or medications were administered.

The composition of whole blood and PRP is presented in Table 2. Preparation of PRP took around 20 min, from the initial blood collection to the final administration.

Table 2. Mean values (±standard deviation) of whole blood and platelet-rich plasma product composition.

Parameter	Whole Blood		Platelet Concentrate	
	Mean Value	SD	Mean Value	SD
Platelets ($\times 10^3/mm^3$)	298.12	78.30	1553.21	400.90
RBC ($\times 10^6/mm^3$)	6.20	1.10	0.50	0.06
WBC ($\times 10^3/mm^3$)	10.16	3.96	4.07	3.09
Lymphocytes ($\times 10^3/mm^3$)	2.05	0.78	2.46	1.63
Monocytes ($\times 10^3/mm^3$)	0.69	0.37	0.52	0.31
Neutrophils ($\times 10^3/mm^3$)	7.03	3.17	0.77	0.32
Eosinophils ($\times 10^3/mm^3$)	0.38	0.43	0.32	0.37
Basophils ($\times 10^3/mm^3$)	0.01	0.02	0.00	0.00

The results of the weight-bearing evaluation and scores of the different client-reported outcome measures in each group are presented in Table 3. No significant differences were observed on day 0. While all treatments produced clinically significant improvements compared to the evaluations on day 0, the combination of PRP and PBMT had greater and longer-lasting effects.

The improvements in PSS and LOAD for each group are presented in Figures 1 and 2, respectively. With the CBPI, a reduction of ≥ 1 in PSS and ≥ 2 in PIS was considered a clinically-important change [41]. The same level has been determined for the LOAD and COI, suggested as a reduction of ≥ 4 and ≥ 14, respectively [42]. Unreported data from our group indicate that clinically important changes consist of improvements of ≥ 1 for deviation and ≥ 10 for SI in dogs with OA.

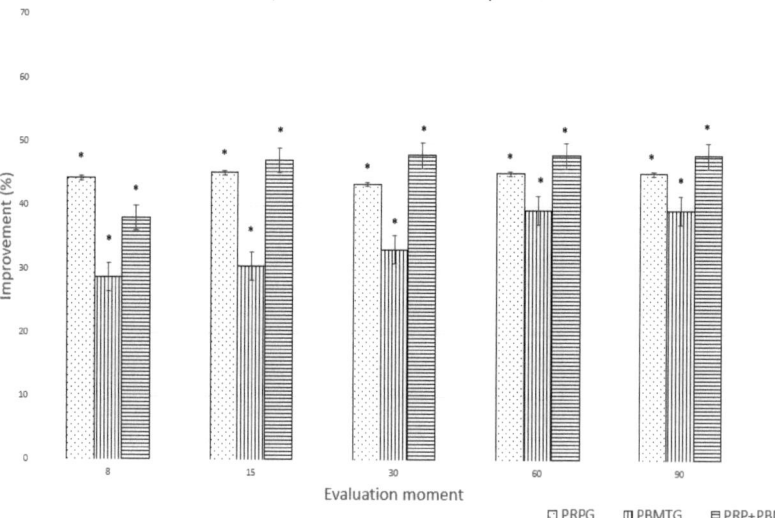

Figure 1. Improvements (%) in Pain Severity Score for the platelet-rich plasma group (PRPG), the photobiomodulation group (PBMTG), and the combined therapies group (PRP+PBMTG), compared to baseline values. * indicates a clinically significant improvement (reduction ≥ 1).

Table 3. Evolution of weight-bearing results and the considered client-reported outcome measures (median, inter-quartile range, and percentual change) by group and moment. CBPI—Canine Brief Pain Inventory; COI—Canine Orthopedic Index; LOAD—Liverpool Osteoarthritis in Dogs; PIS—Pain Interference Score; PSS—Pain Severity Score; QOL—Quality of Life. * indicates significance when comparing groups at each follow-up moment.

Measure		Group	T0			+8 d				+14 d				+30 d				+60 d				+90 d			
			Med	IQR	p	Med	IQR	%	p	Med	IQR	%	p	Med	IQR	%	p	Med	IQR	%	p	Med	IQR	%	p
Weight-bearing	Symmetry Index	PRPG	19.8	40.3	0.85	5.1	5.3	74.1	0.01 *	9.5	5.3	51.8	0.04 *	5.4	13.4	72.6	0.04 *	10.3	24.5	48.2	0.04 *	10.3	24.5	48.2	0.04 *
		PBMTG	20.3	25.3		7.2	13.3	64.5		5.1	5.4	74.7		8.8	12.6	56.6		9.1	12.5	55.1		9.1	12.5	55.1	
		PRP+PBMTG	29.3	26.7		5.3	5.3	82.0		5.0	7.2	82.9		5.3	8.1	82.0		5.1	13.2	82.5		5.1	13.2	82.5	
	Deviation	PRPG	5.5	2.8	0.08	1.0	1.0	81.8	0.24	2.0	1.8	63.6	0.74	1.0	2.3	81.8	0.03 *	3.5	5.5	36.4	0.01 *	3.5	5.5	36.4	0.01 *
		PBMTG	5.0	2.8		2.0	2.8	60.0		2.0	1.0	60.0		3.5	4.5	30.0		4.5	3.8	10.0		4.5	3.8	10.0	
		PRP+PBMTG	6.0	4.5		2.0	1.5	66.7		1.5	1.0	75.0		2.5	4.3	58.3		1.0	3.8	83.3		1.0	3.8	83.3	
CBPI	PSS (0–10)	PRPG	5.3	0.7	0.37	3.0	0.4	44.3	0.71	2.9	0.6	45.1	0.63	3.0	0.8	43.4	0.80	2.9	1.1	45.1	0.76	2.9	1.1	45.1	0.76
		PBMTG	5.1	1.7		3.6	1.7	28.7		3.5	1.7	30.5		3.4	1.9	33.2		3.1	1.8	39.4		3.1	1.8	39.4	
		PRP+PBMTG	5.5	1.0		3.4	0.7	38.0		2.9	1.5	47.1		2.9	1.1	47.9		2.9	1.1	47.9		2.9	1.1	47.9	
	PIS (0–10)	PRPG	4.0	1.0	0.08	1.3	1.3	68.8	0.04 *	1.5	2.3	62.5	0.04 *	1.5	2.4	62.5	0.03 *	2.3	1.8	43.8	0.03 *	2.3	3.3	43.8	0.03 *
		PBMTG	4.5	2.3		2.6	4.8	41.7		4.4	4.8	2.8		2.9	4.1	36.1		2.9	3.6	36.1		2.9	3.6	36.1	
		PRP+PBMTG	5.0	1.7		1.1	2.3	77.5		1.0	4.9	80.0		1.0	3.4	80.0		1.0	1.1	80.0		1.0	1.1	80.0	
LOAD (0–52)		PRPG	20.0	7.5	0.06	13.0	2.0	35.0	0.04 *	13.5	5.3	32.5	0.04 *	13.0	9.5	35.0	0.71	15.5	13.5	22.5	0.81	15.5	13.5	22.5	0.81
		PBMTG	23.5	12.0		16.5	15.3	29.8		17.5	16.8	25.5		16.5	15.5	29.8		13.0	14.3	44.7		13.0	14.3	44.7	
		PRP+PBMTG	26.5	7.0		12.0	3.5	54.7		12.0	15.3	54.7		12.0	10.0	54.7		11.5	11.5	56.6		11.5	11.5	56.6	
COI	Stiffness (0–16)	PRPG	3.2	1.3	0.47	1.5	2.0	53.1	0.04 *	1.4	3.7	56.3	0.04 *	1.5	2.5	53.1	0.03 *	2.6	2.6	18.8	0.03 *	2.6	2.6	18.8	0.03 *
		PBMTG	4.5	2.2		3.0	4.4	33.3		4.3	4.2	4.4		2.6	4.1	42.2		2.7	3.8	40.0		2.7	3.8	40.0	
		PRP+PBMTG	5.0	1.3		1.4	2.7	72.0		1.0	6.0	80.0		1.0	3.3	80.0		1.0	2.0	80.0		1.0	2.0	80.0	
	Function (0–16)	PRPG	7.0	3.8	0.20	4.0	3.8	42.9	0.03 *	4.0	4.8	42.9	0.03 *	4.0	4.0	42.9	0.04 *	4.0	5.3	42.9	0.82	4.0	5.3	42.9	0.82
		PBMTG	6.0	3.5		4.5	5.5	25.0		4.5	16.8	25.0		5.5	5.5	8.3		4.5	6.3	25.0		4.5	6.3	25.0	
		PRP+PBMTG	8.0	0.8		2.5	3.0	68.8		2.0	15.3	75.0		3.5	3.5	56.3		3.0	6.0	62.5		3.0	6.0	62.5	
	Gait (0–20)	PRPG	7.0	3.5	0.54	2.0	2.8	71.4	0.02 *	3.5	3.0	50.0	0.03 *	3.0	2.5	57.1	0.78	4.0	6.0	42.9	0.71	4.0	6.0	42.9	0.71
		PBMTG	6.0	3.8		4.0	6.8	33.3		4.5	6.8	25.0		4.5	6.0	25.0		5.5	6.0	8.3		5.5	6.0	8.3	
		PRP+PBMTG	7.5	1.8		1.0	3.0	86.7		2.5	5.5	66.7		3.5	4.0	53.3		3.5	4.0	53.3		3.5	4.0	53.3	
	QOL (0–12)	PRPG	7.0	2.0	0.71	4.5	3.5	35.7	0.04 *	4.5	7.0	35.7	0.04 *	4.5	4.8	35.7	0.01 *	7.5	8.0	−7.1	0.03 *	7.5	8.0	−7.1	0.03 *
		PBMTG	8.0	5.3		5.5	6.5	31.3		6.0	5.8	25.0		5.0	5.8	37.5		7.0	5.8	12.5		7.0	5.8	12.5	
		PRP+PBMTG	8.0	2.3		2.5	4.5	68.8		2.5	10.0	68.8		3.5	4.0	56.3		3.5	6.3	56.3		3.5	6.3	56.3	
	Overall (0–64)	PRPG	41.0	4.2	0.23	23.5	3.0	42.7	0.03 *	25.5	5.0	37.8	0.01 *	24.5	5.2	40.2	0.01 *	31.0	8.2	24.4	0.04 *	31.0	8.2	24.4	0.04 *
		PBMTG	43.5	6.1		30.5	8.5	29.9		45.5	11.5	−4.6		31.5	8.2	27.6		30.0	8.1	31.0		30.0	8.1	31.0	
		PRP+PBMTG	50.0	2.9		18.0	3.5	64.0		29.0	11.5	42.0		22.5	5.4	55.0		21.5	6.9	57.0		21.5	6.9	57.0	

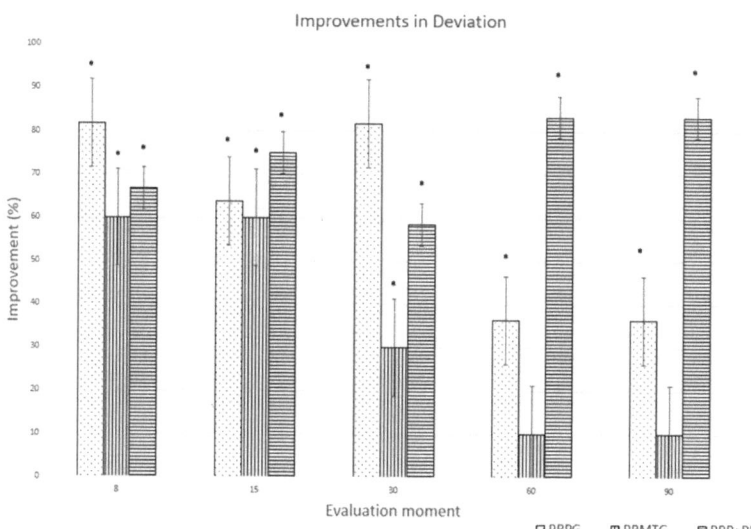

Figure 2. Improvements (%) in deviation in weight-bearing for the platelet-rich plasma group (PRPG), the photobiomodulation group (PBMTG), and the combined therapies group (PRP+PBMTG), compared to baseline values. * indicates a clinically significant improvement (improvement ≥ 1).

4. Discussion

Clinicians usually prefer multimodal approaches in managing OA to cover the multiple dimensions of the disease and to gather the benefits of each therapeutic approach, minimizing possible side effects. Our results show that the combined treatment with PRP and PBMT leads to greater and longer-lasting clinically significant improvements compared to their individual use.

Some reports are available on the individual use of these therapies in managing OA. Regarding intra-articular PRP, many are based on surgically induced models [43–45], but there are also reports available for dogs with naturally occurring OA. As a whole, these products have been able to improve clinical signs at the 12-week evaluation post-treatment or longer [11,46,47]. Our results show that PRP can produce a clinically significant improvement with objective outcome measures and client-reported outcome measures. These improvements lasted until the last evaluation moment, a result in line with the previous report showing a long-lasting therapeutic effect [11].

Similarly, PBMT has been shown to improve pain levels and lameness in dogs with OA alone or in conjunction with NSAID [15,16]. These beneficial effects were observed during treatment but tended to wean out after treatment was discontinued [16]. Our results show that a continued PBMT protocol can improve clinical signs and objective outcome parameters in dogs with hip OA, with long-lasting effects. In fact, pain severity scores showed a continuous improvement over time. It would be interesting to evaluate if this effect persists with time, and future studies should include a longer follow-up period to confirm this finding.

It was interesting to observe that the combined use of PRP and PBMT led to a sustained and consistently greater improvement. At a clinically significant level, this improvement was observed in both objective outcome measures and client-reported outcome measures. A previous report has shown that the concomitant use of PBMT with an NSAID has led to lower doses of NSAID being required to maintain an adequate response to treatment [15]. In our study, lower doses of medication do not apply. Still, improvements are observed with several outcome measures, in many cases from the first follow-up moment and lasting up to the +90 d evaluation. There are several references available reporting that PBMT is commonly employed in conjunction with other treatment modalities for the management of human and animal OA, including therapeutic exercises [48], oral joint supplements [49], and biological treatments [50] that show improved results with the combined therapies. These improvements result from increased downregulation of pro-inflammatory cytokines and metalloproteinases, upregulation of tissue inhibitors of metalloproteinases, and prevention of joint degeneration [50].

The reason for this synergetic effect is not completely clear. Suggested effects of PBMT include stimulation of tissue healing, analgesia, and reduced inflammation [14,51,52]. These effects are attributed to ATP, NO, and reactive oxygen species within cells, altering gene transcription, increasing cell proliferation, and producing growth factors [53]. Similarly, platelets may contribute to tissue regeneration, reduce local inflammation, and to the synthesis of cartilage or inhibition of its breakdown [54], effects mediated by growth factors [55,56]. It is possible that some of the greater improvements are obtained through an increased reduction in inflammation, obtained from the combined use of the two treatment modalities, which act in different pathways. They can also have combined action on inhibiting cartilage breakdown and increasing tissue healing. Another possibility is that PBMT may help improve the degranulation of the platelet's alpha granules or provide a more favorable "field" for liberated growth factors to act. Future studies should include a longer follow-up period to determine if this improvement level is maintained in time.

Although an overall improvement has been observed with most outcome measures considered, improvement with SI and the LOAD seem less remarkable. Some reasons may account for this finding. It has been described that even dogs without OA show some level of asymmetry, up to a 10% level [57]. Although this value was observed with different equipment, a similar phenomenon may be observed with our results. Although it was not a significant difference, a variation in SI was observed between groups at 0 d, but not with deviation. It has been described that dogs with bilateral hip OA can exhibit different compensation mechanisms, even in cases with the same hip OA grade. Some can show side-to-side compensation, while others exhibit pelvic-to-thoracic compensation [34]. This emphasizes the importance of evaluating SI and deviation to obtain an individualized evaluation of each animal evaluation, rather than relying exclusively on expected compensations [41]. With the LOAD, values at the first assessment were relatively low, making it harder to observe a significant improvement. In fact, it has been suggested that including animals with higher client-reported outcome measures scores is preferred, as it increases the likelihood of detecting a clinically significant improvement [27].

We observed some side effects following the intra-articular administration, with some patients showing complaints that resolved without external intervention within 24–72 h. These side effects are similar to those reported following PRP administration, which includes injection pain and local inflammation. They are local, transient, and self-limiting, taking 2–10 days to resolve [58]. We did not record if these complaints were lower in the PRP+PBMT than the PRPG, but this should be evaluated in future studies. Similarly, a power analysis should also be included.

5. Conclusions

This study showed that PRP and PBMT could improve objective outcomes and client-reported outcome measures in dogs with OA. Their combined use leads to greater, longer-lasting, clinically significant improvements. Future studies should address the limitations pointed out in the presented study, including a longer follow-up period to evaluate the duration of the observed improvements in all considered groups and a calculation of power analysis and sample size.

Author Contributions: J.C.A. designed the protocol, conducted treatments, and prepared the manuscript. A.S. selected patients and conducted treatments. L.M.C. revised the protocol and prepared the manuscript. All authors have read and agreed to the published version of the manuscript.

Funding: This research received no external funding.

Institutional Review Board Statement: The study protocol was approved by the ethical review committee of the University of Évora (Órgão Responsável pelo Bem-estar dos Animais da Universidade de Évora, approval no GD/16901/2022).

Informed Consent Statement: Not applicable.

Data Availability Statement: All data generated or analyzed during this study are included in this published article.

Acknowledgments: The authors would like to thank Companion, LLC for donating the PRP systems and Laser equipment used in this study.

Conflicts of Interest: The authors declare that they have no competing interest.

References

1. Alves, J.C.; Santos, A.; Jorge, P.; Lavrador, C.; Carreira, L.M. Clinical and diagnostic imaging findings in police working dogs referred for hip osteoarthritis. *BMC Vet. Res.* **2020**, *16*, 425. [CrossRef] [PubMed]
2. Anderson, K.L.; O'Neill, D.G.; Brodbelt, D.C.; Church, D.B.; Meeson, R.L.; Sargan, D.; Summers, J.F.; Zulch, H.; Collins, L.M. Prevalence, duration and risk factors for appendicular osteoarthritis in a UK dog population under primary veterinary care. *Sci. Rep.* **2018**, *8*, 5641. [CrossRef] [PubMed]
3. Anderson, K.L.; Zulch, H.; O'Neill, D.G.; Meeson, R.L.; Collins, L.M. Risk Factors for Canine Osteoarthritis and Its Predisposing Arthropathies: A Systematic Review. *Front. Vet. Sci.* **2020**, *7*, 220. [CrossRef]
4. Alves, J.C.A.; Jorge, P.I.F.; dos Santos, A.M.M.P. A survey on the orthopedic and functional assessment in a Portuguese population of police working dogs. *BMC Vet. Res.* **2022**, *18*, 116. [CrossRef] [PubMed]
5. Alves, J.C.; Santos, A.; Jorge, P.; Lafuente, P. A multiple-session mesotherapy protocol for the management of hip osteoarthritis in police working dogs. *Am. J. Vet. Res.* **2022**, *84*, 1–8. [CrossRef] [PubMed]
6. Alves, J.C.C.; Santos, A.; Jorge, P.; Lavrador, C.; Carreira, L.M.M. Intraarticular triamcinolone hexacetonide, stanozolol, Hylan G-F 20 and platelet concentrate in a naturally occurring canine osteoarthritis model. *Sci. Rep.* **2021**, *11*, 3118. [CrossRef]
7. Alves, J.C.; Santos, A.; Jorge, P.; Lafuente, P. Multiple session mesotherapy for management of coxofemoral osteoarthritis pain in 10 working dogs: A case series. *Can. Vet. J. Rev. Vet. Can.* **2022**, *63*, 597–602.
8. Alves, J.C.; Santos, A.; Jorge, P.; Lavrador, C.; Carreira, L.M. A report on the use of a single intra-articular administration of autologous platelet therapy in a naturally occurring canine osteoarthritis model—A preliminary study. *BMC Musculoskelet. Disord.* **2020**, *21*, 127. [CrossRef]
9. Alves, J.C.A.; dos Santos, A.M.M.P.; Jorge, P.I.F.; Lavrador, C.F.T.V.B.; Carreira, L.M.A. Management of Osteoarthritis Using 1 Intra-articular Platelet Concentrate Administration in a Canine Osteoarthritis Model. *Am. J. Sports Med.* **2021**, *49*, 599–608. [CrossRef] [PubMed]
10. McDougall, R.A.; Canapp, S.O.; Canapp, D.A. Ultrasonographic Findings in 41 Dogs Treated with Bone Marrow Aspirate Concentrate and Platelet-Rich Plasma for a Supraspinatus Tendinopathy: A Retrospective Study. *Front. Vet. Sci.* **2018**, *5*, 98. [CrossRef]
11. Alves, J.C.; Santos, A.; Jorge, P. Platelet-rich plasma therapy in dogs with bilateral hip osteoarthritis. *BMC Vet. Res.* **2021**, *17*, 207. [CrossRef] [PubMed]
12. Murray, I.R.; Geeslin, A.G.; Goudie, E.B.; Petrigliano, F.A.; LaPrade, R.F. Minimum Information for Studies Evaluating Biologics in Orthopaedics (MIBO). *J. Bone Jt. Surg.* **2017**, *99*, 809–819. [CrossRef] [PubMed]
13. Carr, B.J.; Canapp, S.O.; Mason, D.R.; Cox, C.; Hess, T. Canine Platelet-Rich Plasma Systems: A Prospective Analysis. *Front. Vet. Sci.* **2016**, *2*, 73. [CrossRef] [PubMed]
14. Anders, J.; Kobiela Kertz, A.; Wu, X. Basic principles of photobiomodulation and its effects at the cellular, tissue, and system levels. In *Laser Therapy in Veterinary Medicine: Photobiomodulation*; Riegel, R.J., Goldbold, J., Eds.; Wiley Blackwell: Ames, IA, USA, 2017; pp. 36–52.
15. Looney, A.L.; Huntingford, J.L.; Blaeser, L.L.; Mann, S. A randomized blind placebo-controlled trial investigating the effects of photobiomodulation therapy (PBMT) on canine elbow osteoarthritis. *Can. Vet. J. Rev. Vet. Can.* **2018**, *59*, 959–966.
16. Alves, J.C.; Santos, A.; Jorge, P.; Carreira, L.M. A randomized double-blinded controlled trial on the effects of photobiomodulation therapy in dogs with osteoarthritis. *Am. J. Vet. Res.* **2022**, *83*, ajvr.22.03.0036. [CrossRef]
17. Wardlaw, J.L.; Gazzola, K.M.; Wagoner, A.; Brinkman, E.; Burt, J.; Butler, R.; Gunter, J.M.; Senter, L.H. Laser Therapy for Incision Healing in 9 Dogs. *Front. Vet. Sci.* **2019**, *5*, 349. [CrossRef]
18. Alves, J.C.; Jorge, P.; Santos, A. The effect of photobiomodulation therapy on the management of chronic idiopathic large-bowel diarrhea in dogs. *Lasers Med. Sci.* **2021**, *97*, 2045–2051. [CrossRef]
19. Alves, J.C.; Jorge, P.; Santos, A. The Effect of Photobiomodulation Therapy on Inflammation Following Dental Prophylaxis. *J. Vet. Dent.* **2023**, 089875642211505. [CrossRef]
20. Lascelles, B.D.X.; Roe, S.C.; Smith, E.; Reynolds, L.; Markham, J.; Marcellin-Little, D.; Bergh, M.S.; Budsberg, S.C. Evaluation of a pressure walkway system for measurement of vertical limb forces in clinically normal dogs. *Am. J. Vet. Res.* **2006**, *67*, 277–282. [CrossRef]

21. Hyytiäinen, H.K.; Mölsä, S.H.; Junnila, J.T.; Laitinen-Vapaavuori, O.M.; Hielm-Björkman, A.K. Use of bathroom scales in measuring asymmetry of hindlimb static weight bearing in dogs with osteoarthritis. *Vet. Comp. Orthop. Traumatol.* **2012**, *25*, 390–396. [CrossRef]
22. Seibert, R.; Marcellin-Little, D.J.; Roe, S.C.; DePuy, V.; Lascelles, B.D.X. Comparison of Body Weight Distribution, Peak Vertical Force, and Vertical Impulse as Measures of Hip Joint Pain and Efficacy of Total Hip Replacement. *Vet. Surg.* **2012**, *41*, 443–447. [CrossRef]
23. Clough, W.; Canapp, S.; Taboada, L.; Dycus, D.; Leasure, C. Sensitivity and specificity of a weight distribution platform for the detection of objective lameness and orthopaedic disease. *Vet. Comp. Orthop. Traumatol.* **2018**, *31*, 391–395. [CrossRef]
24. Clough, W.; Canapp, S. Assessing clinical relevance of weight distribution as measured on a stance analyzer through comparison with lameness determined on a pressure sensitive walkway and clinical diagnosis. *Vet. Comp. Orthop. Traumatol.* **2018**, *31*, A1–A25. [CrossRef]
25. Albuquerque, N.; Guo, K.; Wilkinson, A.; Savalli, C.; Otta, E.; Mills, D. Dogs recognize dog and human emotions. *Biol. Lett.* **2016**, *12*, 20150883. [CrossRef] [PubMed]
26. Wiseman-Orr, M.L.; Nolan, A.M.; Reid, J.; Scott, E.M. Development of a questionnaire to measure the effects of chronic pain on health-related quality of life in dogs. *Am. J. Vet. Res.* **2004**, *65*, 1077–1084. [CrossRef] [PubMed]
27. Walton, B.; Cox, T.; Innes, J. 'How do I know my animal got better?'—Measuring outcomes in small animal orthopaedics. *Practice* **2018**, *40*, 42–50. [CrossRef]
28. Walton, M.B.; Cowderoy, E.; Lascelles, D.; Innes, J.F. Evaluation of construct and criterion validity for the 'Liverpool Osteoarthritis in Dogs' (LOAD) clinical metrology instrument and comparison to two other instruments. *PLoS ONE* **2013**, *8*, e58125. [CrossRef]
29. Brown, D.C. The Canine Orthopedic Index. Step 2: Psychometric testing. *Vet. Surg.* **2014**, *43*, 241–246. [CrossRef]
30. Brown, D.C.; Boston, R.C.; Coyne, J.C.; Farrar, J.T. Ability of the canine brief pain inventory to detect response to treatment in dogs with osteoarthritis. *J. Am. Vet. Med. Assoc.* **2008**, *233*, 1278–1283. [CrossRef] [PubMed]
31. Radke, H.; Joeris, A.; Chen, M. Evidence-based evaluation of owner-reported outcome measures for canine orthopedic care—A COSMIN evaluation of 6 instruments. *Vet. Surg.* **2022**, *51*, 244–253. [CrossRef] [PubMed]
32. Monteiro, B.P.; Lascelles, B.D.X.; Murrell, J.; Robertson, S.; Steagall, P.V.M.; Wright, B. 2022 WSAVA guidelines for the recognition, assessment and treatment of pain. *J. Small Anim. Pract.* **2023**, *64*, 177–254. [CrossRef]
33. Flückiger, M. Scoring Radiographs for Canine Hip Dysplasia—The Big Three Organisations in the World. *Eur. J. Compagnion Anim. Pract.* **2008**, *2*, 135–140.
34. Alves, J.C.; Santos, A.; Jorge, P.; Lavrador, C.; Carreira, L.M. Characterization of Weight-bearing Compensation in Dogs with Bilateral Hip Osteoarthritis. *Top. Companion Anim. Med.* **2022**, *49*, 100655. [CrossRef]
35. Volstad, N.; Sandberg, G.; Robb, S.; Budsberg, S. The evaluation of limb symmetry indices using ground reaction forces collected with one or two force plates in healthy dogs. *Vet. Comp. Orthop. Traumatol.* **2017**, *30*, 54–58. [CrossRef]
36. Alves, J.C.; Santos, A.; Jorge, P. Initial psychometric evaluation of the Portuguese version of the Canine Brief Pain Inventory. *Am. J. Vet. Res.* **2022**, *84*, 1–6. [CrossRef]
37. Alves, J.C.; Jorge, P.; Santos, A. Initial psychometric evaluation of the Portuguese version of the Liverpool Osteoarthritis in Dogs. *BMC Vet. Res.* **2022**, *18*, 367. [CrossRef]
38. Alves, J.C. Initial Psychometric Evaluation of the Portuguese Version of the Canine Orthopedic Index. *Vet. Comp. Orthop. Traumatol.* **2023**, *36*, 236–240. [CrossRef]
39. Alves, J.C.; Santos, A.; Jorge, P.; Lavrador, C.; Carreira, L.M. Evaluation of Four Clinical Metrology Instruments for the Assessment of Osteoarthritis in Dogs. *Animals* **2022**, *12*, 2808. [CrossRef] [PubMed]
40. Laflamme, D. Development and validation of a body condition score system for dogs. *Canine Pract.* **1997**, *22*, 10–15.
41. Brown, D.C.; Bell, M.; Rhodes, L. Power of treatment success definitions when the Canine Brief Pain Inventory is used to evaluate carprofen treatment for the control of pain and inflammation in dogs with osteoarthritis. *Am. J. Vet. Res.* **2013**, *74*, 1467–1473. [CrossRef]
42. Innes, J.F.; Morton, M.A.; Lascelles, B.D.X. Minimal clinically-important differences for the 'Liverpool Osteoarthritis in Dogs' (LOAD) and the 'Canine Orthopedic Index' (COI) client-reported outcomes measures. *PLoS ONE* **2023**, *18*, e0280912. [CrossRef]
43. Vilar, J.M.; Manera, M.E.; Santana, A.; Spinella, G.; Rodriguez, O.; Rubio, M.; Carrillo, J.M.; Sopena, J.; Batista, M. Effect of leukocyte-reduced platelet-rich plasma on osteoarthritis caused by cranial cruciate ligament rupture: A canine gait analysis model. *PLoS ONE* **2018**, *13*, e0194752. [CrossRef] [PubMed]
44. Lee, M.-I.; Kim, J.-H.; Kwak, H.-H.; Woo, H.-M.; Han, J.-H.; Yayon, A.; Jung, Y.-C.; Cho, J.-M.; Kang, B.-J. A placebo-controlled study comparing the efficacy of intra-articular injections of hyaluronic acid and a novel hyaluronic acid-platelet-rich plasma conjugate in a canine model of osteoarthritis. *J. Orthop. Surg. Res.* **2019**, *14*, 314. [CrossRef] [PubMed]
45. Yun, S.; Ku, S.-K.; Kwon, Y.-S. Adipose-derived mesenchymal stem cells and platelet-rich plasma synergistically ameliorate the surgical-induced osteoarthritis in Beagle dogs. *J. Orthop. Surg. Res.* **2016**, *11*, 9. [CrossRef]
46. Fahie, M.A.; Ortolano, G.A.; Guercio, V.; Schaffer, J.A.; Johnston, G.; Au, J.; Hettlich, B.A.; Phillips, T.; Allen, M.J.; Bertone, A.L. A randomized controlled trial of the efficacy of autologous platelet therapy for the treatment of osteoarthritis in dogs. *J. Am. Vet. Med. Assoc.* **2013**, *243*, 1291–1297. [CrossRef]

47. Cuervo, B.; Chicharro, D.; Del Romero, A.; Damia, E.; Carrillo, J.; Sopena, J.; Peláez, P.; Miguel, L.; Vilar, J.; Rubio, M. Objective and subjective evaluation of plasma rich in growth factors therapy for the treatment of osteoarthritis in dogs. *Osteoarthr. Cartil.* **2019**, *27*, S482. [CrossRef]
48. Vassão, P.G.; Parisi, J.; Penha, T.F.C.; Balão, A.B.; Renno, A.C.M.; Avila, M.A. Association of photobiomodulation therapy (PBMT) and exercises programs in pain and functional capacity of patients with knee osteoarthritis (KOA): A systematic review of randomized trials. *Lasers Med. Sci.* **2021**, *36*, 1341–1353. [CrossRef] [PubMed]
49. Sanches, M.; Assis, L.; Criniti, C.; Fernandes, D.; Tim, C.; Renno, A.C.M. Chondroitin sulfate and glucosamine sulfate associated to photobiomodulation prevents degenerative morphological changes in an experimental model of osteoarthritis in rats. *Lasers Med. Sci.* **2018**, *33*, 549–557. [CrossRef] [PubMed]
50. Stancker, T.G.; Vieira, S.S.; Serra, A.J.; do Nascimento Lima, R.; dos Santos Feliciano, R.; Silva, J.A.; dos Santos, S.A.; dos Santos Vieira, M.A.; Simões, M.C.B.; Leal-Junior, E.C.; et al. Can photobiomodulation associated with implantation of mesenchymal adipose-derived stem cells attenuate the expression of MMPs and decrease degradation of type II collagen in an experimental model of osteoarthritis? *Lasers Med. Sci.* **2018**, *33*, 1073–1084. [CrossRef] [PubMed]
51. Villela, P.A.; de Souza, N.D.C.; Baia, J.D.; Gioso, M.A.; Aranha, A.C.C.; de Freitas, P.M. Antimicrobial photodynamic therapy (aPDT) and photobiomodulation (PBM—660 nm) in a dog with chronic gingivostomatitis. *Photodiagn. Photodyn. Ther.* **2017**, *20*, 273–275. [CrossRef]
52. Watson, A.H.; Brundage, C.M. Photobiomodulation as an Inflammatory Therapeutic Following Dental Prophylaxis in Canines. *Photobiomodul. Photomed. Laser Surg.* **2019**, *37*, 276–281. [CrossRef]
53. Kennedy, K.C.; Martinez, S.A.; Martinez, S.E.; Tucker, R.L.; Davies, N.M. Effects of low-level laser therapy on bone healing and signs of pain in dogs following tibial plateau leveling osteotomy. *Am. J. Vet. Res.* **2018**, *79*, 893–904. [CrossRef]
54. Fukui, N.; Purple, C.R.; Sandell, L.J. Cell biology of osteoarthritis: The chondrocyte's response to injury. *Curr. Rheumatol. Rep.* **2001**, *3*, 496–505. [CrossRef]
55. Cole, B.J.; Seroyer, S.T.; Filardo, G.; Bajaj, S.; Fortier, L.A. Platelet-rich plasma: Where are we now and where are we going? *Sport. Health A Multidiscip. Approach* **2010**, *2*, 203–210. [CrossRef] [PubMed]
56. Nguyen, R.T.; Borg-Stein, J.; McInnis, K. Applications of platelet-rich plasma in musculoskeletal and Sports Medicine: An evidence-based approach. *PM&R* **2011**, *3*, 226–250. [CrossRef]
57. Brønniche Møller Nielsen, M.; Pedersen, T.; Mouritzen, A.; Vitger, A.D.; Nielsen, L.N.; Poulsen, H.H.; Miles, J.E. Kinetic gait analysis in healthy dogs and dogs with osteoarthritis: An evaluation of precision and overlap performance of a pressure-sensitive walkway and the use of symmetry indices. *PLoS ONE* **2020**, *15*, e0243819. [CrossRef]
58. Ornetti, P.; Nourissat, G.; Berenbaum, F.; Sellam, J.; Richette, P.; Chevalier, X. Does platelet-rich plasma have a role in the treatment of osteoarthritis? *Jt. Bone Spine* **2016**, *83*, 31–36. [CrossRef]

Disclaimer/Publisher's Note: The statements, opinions and data contained in all publications are solely those of the individual author(s) and contributor(s) and not of MDPI and/or the editor(s). MDPI and/or the editor(s) disclaim responsibility for any injury to people or property resulting from any ideas, methods, instructions or products referred to in the content.

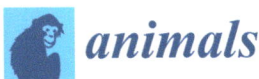

Article

Bacterial Contamination of Environmental Surfaces of Veterinary Rehabilitation Clinics

Henry G. Spratt [1],*, Nicholas Millis [2], David Levine [3], Jenna Brackett [1] and Darryl Millis [2]

[1] Department of Biology, Geology, and Environmental Science, University of Tennessee at Chattanooga, Chattanooga, TN 37403, USA; jennabrac@gmail.com
[2] Department of Small Animal Clinical Sciences, University of Tennessee College of Veterinary Medicine, Knoxville, TN 37996, USA; nickmillis1996@gmail.com (N.M.); boneplate@aol.com (D.M.)
[3] Department of Physical Therapy, University of Tennessee at Chattanooga, Chattanooga, TN 37403, USA; david-levine@utc.edu
* Correspondence: henry-spratt@utc.edu; Tel.: +1-423-425-4383

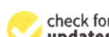

Citation: Spratt, H.G.; Millis, N.; Levine, D.; Brackett, J.; Millis, D. Bacterial Contamination of Environmental Surfaces of Veterinary Rehabilitation Clinics. *Animals* **2024**, *14*, 1896. https://doi.org/10.3390/ani14131896

Academic Editors: L. Miguel Carreira and João Alves

Received: 30 April 2024
Revised: 20 June 2024
Accepted: 25 June 2024
Published: 27 June 2024

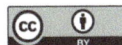

Copyright: © 2024 by the authors. Licensee MDPI, Basel, Switzerland. This article is an open access article distributed under the terms and conditions of the Creative Commons Attribution (CC BY) license (https://creativecommons.org/licenses/by/4.0/).

Simple Summary: This study was conducted to provide background data on the potential bacterial contamination of environmental surfaces in veterinary rehabilitation clinics. Knowledge of bacterial contamination in these clinics is important for effective rehabilitative outcomes for veterinary patients. This is particularly true when surgery has occurred prior to the rehabilitation. There is abundant evidence from human surgical recovery and rehabilitation that surgical site infections (SSIs) represent a major type of healthcare-associated infection. With human patients, *Staphylococcus* spp. (including the methicillin *S. aureus* strain—MRSA) are often associated with SSIs. For human patients, SSIs have been correlated with environmental bacterial contamination in clinics. Whether SSIs in veterinary patients are more prevalent when clinic environments are contaminated with potentially pathogenic bacteria has not been the subject of any substantial research to date. The purpose of this study is to provide background data on presumptive environmental surface bacterial contamination by potential pathogens in veterinary rehabilitation clinics. Our data suggest that bacterial contamination in these clinics is widespread. We have detected potential pathogens, including MRSA, *S. pseudintermedius*, various enteric bacteria, and *Clostridium difficile*, in the clinics sampled. These bacterial species may pose a problem to either clinic veterinary patients or human caregivers.

Abstract: The presence of potentially pathogenic bacteria on veterinary clinic surfaces may be problematic. In this study, we collected swab samples (Fisherbrand, double transport swabs with Stuart's liquid medium) and water samples from five veterinary rehabilitation clinics. Swabs and water samples were transported to a microbiology lab for processing. At the lab, swabs were used to inoculate Hardy's Cdiff Banana Broth (for *Clostridium difficile* [Cdiff]) and five different types of bacterial growth media, including Hardy CHROM MRSA agar (methicillin-resistant *Staphylococcus aureus* [MRSA] and *S. pseudintermedius* [SIM]), mannitol salt agar (*S. aureus* [SA]), eosin methylene blue agar (enterics [ENT]), *Pseudomonas* isolation agar (*Pseudomonas* spp. [PS]), and tryptic soy agar [TSA] (non-specific). The most prominent presumptive species cultured was Cdiff (on nearly 55% of swabs). *Bacillus* spp. and enteric bacteria were encountered on nearly 35% of swabs, with MRSA and SIM on just over 10% of swabs. The most contaminated sample site was harnesses/life jackets used with the underwater treadmill (33% of swabs). The underwater treadmill water had total bacterial counts from 1600 to 2800 cfu/mL. Of all presumptive bacterial species detected, SIM tends to be more pathogenic for dogs. Targeted cleaning/disinfecting in these clinics could help reduce risks for both animals and caregivers utilizing these clinics.

Keywords: veterinary rehabilitation; canine rehabilitation; bacterial contamination; clinic environmental surfaces; staphylococci; MRSA; *Clostridium difficile*

1. Introduction

Healthcare-associated infections (HAIs) are a concern for patients treated in medical facilities, including veterinary physical rehabilitation facilities [1–3]. Pathogens can be especially concerning for postoperative patients or those who are hospitalized for prolonged time periods. These concerns are important in facilities for human and animal patients, with potential transmission from equipment or other external surfaces to the patients as a possible cause of HAIs [4,5]. In human medicine, certain pathogens tend to be of the most concern for serious medical problems, including *Clostridium difficile* [Cdiff], *Staphylococcus aureus* ([SA], especially methicillin-resistant variants [e.g., MRSA]), *Staphylococcus pseudintermedius* [SIM], and multidrug-resistant, Gram-negative rods (e.g., enteric bacteria [ENT] that may include *Escherichia* spp., *Enterobacter* sp. and *Klebsiella* sp.). While not necessarily of equal concern in human and veterinary clinics, the presence of these bacterial species on surfaces in any clinic represents contamination that could lead to HAIs [6].

Veterinary rehabilitation clinics represent a specialty of veterinary medicine in which animals that are recovering from an injury or surgery receive rehabilitation similar to human physical therapy. These rehabilitation clinics include therapeutic modalities, such as therapeutic ultrasound and lasers [7], and exercise equipment, such as treadmills, underwater treadmills, therapy balls, and other unstable surfaces for exercise [8]. These clinics commonly see postoperative patients with healing incisions and animals that are paralyzed or have limited mobility. Avoiding the contamination of surgical site wounds and preventing infections from shared equipment is important to consider in veterinary rehabilitation.

The bacterial contamination of surfaces in veterinary rehabilitation clinics can be problematic for both the animals being treated and the human caretakers. For example, Cdiff is a pathogen that can cause severe disease in humans. Infection by Cdiff can cause severe diarrhea and pseudomembranous colitis [9,10]. Although Cdiff has been isolated from dogs, a link between human infection with Cdiff and companion animals is not well documented and should be further explored [11–13].

Staphylococci, including SA and SIM, are opportunistic pathogens in both humans and animals [14–17]. Typically, SA infections have been successfully treated with topical or systemic courses of antibiotics [15]. However, antibiotic-resistant staphylococcal strains, including MRSA, represent an increasing problem throughout all of healthcare. These pathogens may also be isolated from companion animal veterinary patients, in addition to other pathogens that affect animals, and can also be transmitted from humans to animals.

Pathogens with known transmission between humans and animals include SA, MRSA, and SIM [16,17]. Orden et al. [11] isolated Cdiff from 12% of the dogs they studied. In a similar study, Álvarez-Perez et al. [6] found Cdiff infections in 5% of the dogs they sampled. Cdiff can cause enteritis, diarrhea, and hemorrhagic diarrhea in both humans and dogs [11,18]. Since Cdiff can be isolated from dogs, a major concern is the possible transfer of this pathogen to human caregivers. Since Cdiff spores may be found on the environmental surfaces of both human and animal clinics, knowledge of this contamination in veterinary clinics could be important to prevent HAIs in both humans and animals.

Staphylococcal infections in canine patients are often the result of surgical procedures and may cause moderate to severe morbidity [19]. With the continued impact of MRSA in human medicine and the close contact between humans and household pets, there has been an increase in MRSA in household pets [20]. Most infections associated with MRSA in veterinary patients are community-acquired and often transmitted from pet owners to their pets [21]. The prevalence of MRSA infections in veterinary patients ranges from 0 to 9% and may result in different symptoms related to skin and soft tissue infections, especially surgical site wounds, otitis, and pyoderma [15,21,22].

Staphylococcus pseudintermedius is a more common form of *Staphylococcus* spp. isolated from dogs and is responsible for infections such as pyoderma and otitis [23,24]. Starting in 2005, *S. pseudintermedius* became a novel species within the *S. intermedius* group of staphylococci [25]. It was formerly believed that dogs were colonized by *S. intermedius*, but in fact, the most common staphylococcal opportunistic pathogen associated with dogs is

S. pseudintermedius [26–28]. Similar to other *Staphylococcus* spp. isolates, *S. pseudintermedius* causes urinary tract infections, otitis, wound infection, soft tissue infections, and surgical site infections and is the leading cause of pyoderma in dogs [29,30]. Similar to strains of SA, *S. pseudintermedius* has developed resistance to methicillin, resulting in more complex and costly treatment options for veterinary patients [4,11,31]. It is known that the spread of *S. pseudintermedius* usually involves contact between two hosts. With increased exposure between humans and veterinary patients, the risk of the transmission of pathogens will likely rise, especially with MRSA, antibiotic-resistant SIM, and Cdiff [12,21,32]. Zoonotic pathogens are a huge public health concern, and interspecies transfer of these pathogens between animals and humans could enhance the horizontal exchange of resistance factors between these pathogens [12,21,32].

With the close contact between pets and their owners, other animal patients, and veterinary medical personnel in veterinary rehabilitation facilities, it is important to know if surfaces within the facility are contaminated by potential pathogens. Knowledge of problematic surface spots in these clinics should encourage managers of these clinics to proactively clean and disinfect sites known to be contaminated by these pathogens. The aim of this study was to determine the prevalence of contamination by potential pathogens of both humans and animals from environmental surfaces and equipment commonly found in veterinary physical rehabilitation clinics. Overall, we found bacterial contamination by potential pathogens to be commonplace throughout the clinics sampled. Future studies should seek any links between this background contamination and the incidence of HAIs in clinic patients.

2. Materials and Methods

This study involved the collection of bacterial swab samples from environmental surfaces and water samples from underwater treadmill tanks in five different veterinary rehabilitation clinics. Within the clinics, we identified 13 items/locations (Table 1) that were present in each clinic for the collection of swab samples. Sampling involved using double transport swabs (Fisherbrand, with Stuart's liquid medium, Fisher Scientific, Pittsburg, PA, USA), which were used to sample areas of approximately 100 cm^2 at each sample site. Both of the two swabs present in these double swabs were carefully brought into contact with the surfaces sampled. For additional information regarding how these swabs were used to inoculate growth medium and how the surface areas of the swabs were estimated, please see the Supplementary Materials File S1. After collection, the swabs were placed on ice and transported to a microbiology lab on the University of Tennessee at Chattanooga (UTC) campus for processing (within four hours of swab collection). This lab is a Biosafety Level 2 certified lab, all personnel working with the samples wore appropriate personal protection equipment (e.g., lab coat, safety glasses, and gloves), and all swab and culture manipulations occurred in a properly functioning biosafety cabinet.

Table 1. Percentage of positive swabs having viable bacteria by site and bacterial type or species. Legend: UWTM = underwater treadmill; exercise equipment = peanuts, balance boards, physiorolls, donuts, etc.; MRSA = methicillin-resistant *S. aureus*, SA = *S. aureus*, SE = *S. epidermidis* (mannitol-negative), SIM = *S. pseudintermedius*, ENT = enteric bacteria (lactose-positive, Gram-negative rods), PS = *Pseudomonas* spp., PSA = *P. aeruginosa*, ML = *Micrococcus* spp., BAC = *Bacillus* spp., Cdiff = *Clostridium difficile*.

	MRSA	SA	SE	SIM	ENT	PS	PSA	ML	BAC	Cdiff
Dry Treadmill (belt, n = 5)	40%	40%	40%	0%	40%	0%	0%	100%	60%	80%
Exercise Equipment (n = 27)	11.1%	18.5%	22.2%	0%	25.9%	11.1%	0%	22.2%	44.4%	74.1%
Floors (n = 19)	15.8%	52.6%	31.6%	15.8%	52.6%	31.6%	5.3%	21.1%	63.2%	94.7%
Harnesses (n = 8)	0%	25%	12.5%	25%	12.5%	0%	0%	12.5%	12.5%	75%
Laser Probes (tip of probe, n = 9)	0%	11.1%	11.1%	11.1%	11.1%	0%	0%	0%	0%	33.3%
Life Jackets (n = 10)	0%	0%	30%	10%	40%	10%	0%	40%	10%	60%
Return Air Ducts (n = 6)	15.8%	83.3%	33.3%	16.7%	100%	16.7%	0%	16.7%	100%	16.7%
Scales (n = 6)	50%	83.3%	33.3%	33.3%	83.3%	16.7%	16.7%	16.7%	100%	66.7%

Table 1. Cont.

	MRSA	SA	SE	SIM	ENT	PS	PSA	ML	BAC	Cdiff
Ultrasound Gel (bottle tip, n = 4)	0%	0%	50%	0%	0%	0%	0%	0%	0%	25%
Ultrasound Heads (n = 6)	0%	0%	0%	0%	0%	0%	0%	0%	16.7%	16.7%
UWTM Top Belt (n = 7)	14.3%	14.3%	14.3%	14.3%	14.3%	14.3%	0%	28.6%	28.6%	28.6%
UWTM Bottom Surface of Belt (n = 7)	0%	0%	0%	0%	0%	0%	0%	0%	0%	28.6%
UWTM Jets (inside surface) (n = 8)	0%	0%	12.5%	12.5%	50%	25%	25%	12.5%	25%	12.5%

At the lab, these swabs were used to inoculate four different selective and differential media types, one selective enrichment broth, and one non-specific bacterial growth medium. The media used included two from Hardy Diagnostics (Hardy Diagnostics, Santa Maria, CA, USA), as follows: a selective enrichment broth, Hardy Cdiff Banana Broth (Hardy Cat.# K226, selective for the enrichment of Clostridium difficile [Cdiff]), and a selective and differential agar, Hardy Diagnostic's CHROM MRSA agar (Hardy Cat.# G307, selective for methicillin-resistant *S. aureus* [MRSA] and *S. pseudintermedius* [SIM]). We used three selective and differential medium agars from Fisher Scientific (Fisher Scientific, Pittsburgh, PA, USA), including mannitol salt agar (Fisher Cat.# B2127X [BD Mfr.# 221271] for *S. aureus* [SA] and *S. epidermidis* [SE]); eosin methylene blue agar (Fisher Cat.#. B11221 [BD Mfr.# 211221], EMB, for enteric bacteria [ENT]); and pseudomonas isolation agar (Fisher Cat.# DF0927-17-1 [BD Mfr.# 292710] for *Pseudomonas* spp. [PS] and *P. aeruginosa* [PSA]). In addition to the selective and differential media, we also inoculated a non-specific type of bacterial growth media, tryptic soy agar [TSA] (Fisher Cat.# DF0369-17-6 [BD Mfr.# 236950]), which was used to detect *Bacillus* spp. [BAC] and *Micrococcus* spp. [ML]. The inoculation of the Hardy Cdiff banana broth necessitated the use of one of the two double swabs, with that swab being aseptically transferred into the broth tube and clipped off with flame-sterilized scissors to allow the swab to fit inside the tube. The second of the double swabs was then used to inoculate all the selective and differential media and the TSA plates using a line inoculation technique (as described in Keilman et al. [33], please see the Supplementary Materials for more information regarding this line inoculation technique). In short, for the line inoculations, the five agar plates to be inoculated were placed side by side in the biosafety cabinet, and using a gentle, short, 4 cm, straight-line motion, one medium at a time was inoculated. When changing to a new agar type, the swab shafts were rotated approximately 1/5 of a rotation to bring a fresh surface of the swab to the different agar surfaces. Inoculated agar plates and the Hardy banana broth tubes were placed in a 37 °C incubator and incubated for 48 h.

Water samples were collected from the underwater treadmill tanks using a 10 mL pipette with sterile pipette tips, transferring these samples into sterile WhirlPack sample bags (500 mL, Fisher Scientific, Pittsburgh, PA, USA), and after proper sealing, all the sample bags were placed in a cooler on ice for transport back to the microbiology lab at UTC. At the lab, 0.1 mL subsamples were aseptically removed from the sample bags using pipettes with sterile tips and transferred onto the surface of TSA and EMB plates. These aliquots of water samples were spread over the entire surface of the plates using flame-sterilized spreading rods. Plates inoculated with water samples were also placed in a 37 °C incubator and incubated for 48 h.

The interpretation of bacterial growth on the different media allowed for the observation of different types of bacteria colonies typically found to grow on the specific medium types, leading to our presumptive conclusions. For additional information regarding how different presumptive bacterial identifications were made from incubated media, please see the Supplementary Materials. We were also able to count the number of colonies growing on the plates inoculated with water samples. For the selective and differential media used to indicate staphylococci presence, growth on MSA enabled the detection of both mannitol-positive (for fermentation, turning the medium yellow with white to tan colonies, e.g., SA) staphylococci and mannitol-negative staphylococci (with white colonies leaving the medium red, e.g., SE). Using the CHROM MRSA agar plates, mauve-colored to white with pink streak colonies were known to represent presumptive colonies of MRSA [34]. Using EMB agar plates, pink to dark purple colonies were indicative of lactose fermentation and were used to presumptively identify enteric bacteria [ENT]. For *Pseudomonas* spp. we scored yellowish-green colonies on PSI agar as positive for *P. aeruginosa* [PSA] and white colonies as *Pseudomonas* spp. [PS]. Colonies growing on the TSA plates were used to estimate the overall level of non-specific bacterial colonization of the different sites sampled, specifically allowing for the observation of *Bacillus* spp. [BAC]. or *Micrococcus* spp. [ML].

Once bacterial identification on the plates was determined, these data were presented as percent-positive swabs by species and sample site. Data were analyzed using descriptive statistics. The analysis was performed using SPSS 26 (Armonk, NY, USA: IBM Corp).

3. Results

The most common presumptive contaminating species based on an average of percent-positive swabs for all sites was Cdiff, with BAC and ENT being the next two most common contaminating bacterial types observed. Contamination by Cdiff was found at 58.3% of all sites sampled, while BAC and ENT were found on 35.4% and 33.1% of sites (Figure 1). At the lower end of the contamination range, we found PSA contaminating only 3.6% of sites.

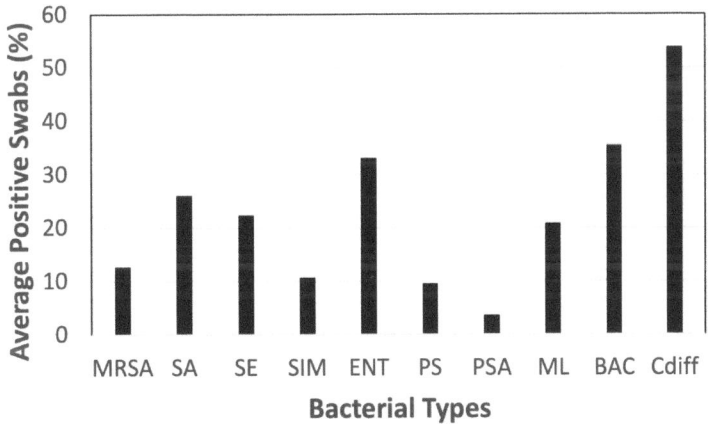

Figure 1. Average of the percent-positive swabs for all sites by bacterial species. Key: MRSA = methicillin-resistant *S. aureus*, SA = *S. aureus*, SE = *S. epidermidis* (mannitol-negative), SIM = *S. pseudintermedius*, ENT = enteric bacteria (lactose-positive, Gram-negative rods), PS = *Pseudomonas* spp., PSA = *P. aeruginosa*, ML = *Micrococcus* spp., BAC = *Bacillus* spp., Cdiff = *Clostridium difficile*.

When looking at clinic contamination by site and species, Cdiff contaminated 94.7% of the floors and 83.3% of the HVAC return air ducts (Table 1). Enteric bacteria and *Bacillus* spp. were the next most encountered contaminants and were found on 100% of swabs from the return air ducts. The floors and return air ducts were consistently contaminated by other species, including Cdiff, SA, MRSA, and SIM. The highest levels of contamination by SA were found on the HVAC return air duct (83.3%) and the scales (83.3%).

When looking at the presumptive bacterial contamination of different clinic sites, a large range of contamination was observed. Staphylococci were found most prominently on the floors, with SA found on the largest number of swabs (Figure 2). The only sites in which staphylococci were not found were the ultrasound gel bottles and heads and the bottom surface of the belt on the underwater treadmills.

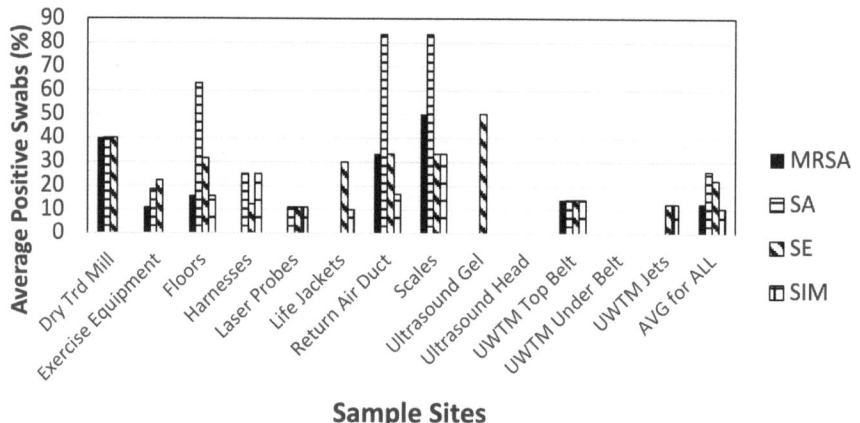

Figure 2. Total positive swabs by site having *Staphylococcus* spp. Presumptive species identification: MRSA = methicillin-resistant *S. aureus*, SA = *S. aureus*, SE = *S. epidermidis*, SIM = *S. pseudintermedius*.

Bacterial contamination due to select Gram-negative rods was also found throughout the veterinary clinics. Enteric bacterial contamination (lactose-positive cells, e.g., *Escherichia* spp.) was found on the greatest number of sampled sites of the Gram-negative bacteria studied (Figure 3). Again, the floors were the most contaminated sites in these clinics. *Pseudomonas aeruginosa* was also found in the clinics, but in relatively low numbers. Other species of *Pseudomonas* spp. were generally widespread in the clinics at slightly higher numbers.

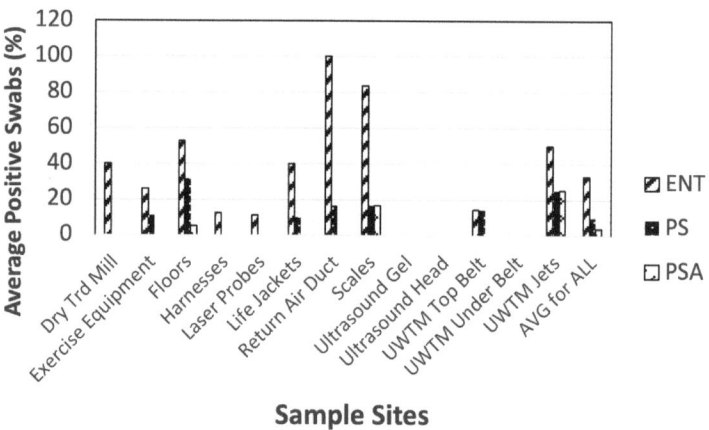

Figure 3. Total positive swabs by site with select Gram-negative bacteria. Presumptive species identification: ENT = enteric bacteria (lactose-positive, e.g., *Escherichia* spp.), PS = *Pseudomonas* spp., PSA = *Pseudomonas aeruginosa*.

Bacterial contamination by other select Gram-positive species was also found throughout the clinics. Most notably, Cdiff was found in a very high number of sites throughout the clinics (Figure 4). Another spore-forming genera of Gram-positive bacteria, *Bacillus* sp., was also found contaminating many of the same sites as Cdiff. *Micrococcus* spp., a Gram-positive coccus often associated with human skin, was also found on many sites throughout the clinic.

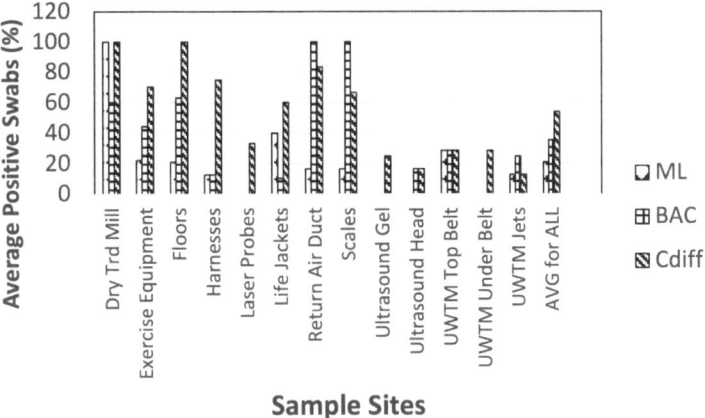

Figure 4. Total positive swabs by site with select Gram-positive bacteria. Presumptive species identification: ML = *Micrococcus* spp., BAC = *Bacillus* spp., Cdiff = *Clostridium difficile*.

When water from underwater treadmill tanks was streaked onto TSA and EMB agar plates, colony counts as high as 2800 cfu/mL were detected (Figure 5). The largest number of bacterial colonies observed was for enteric bacteria.

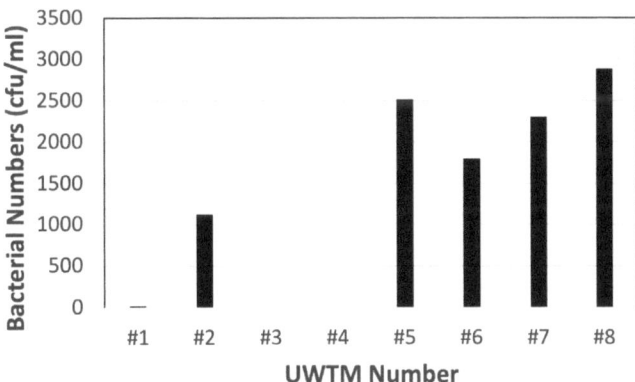

Figure 5. Water sample contamination for water from underwater treadmill (UWTM) tanks at five veterinary clinic sites. Individual UWTMs are indicated by number (#1 through #4 were at one clinic, while #5 to #8 were each at different clinics). Total colony counts (per mL) for TSA and EMB media streaked with 0.1 mL samples from the treadmill tanks.

4. Discussion

This study assessed the patterns of bacterial contamination on medical equipment and environmental sites in veterinary physical rehabilitation clinics. Bacterial species that were isolated and grown included both Gram-negative and Gram-positive bacteria. Of the Gram-positive cocci, several *Staphylococcus* spp. were observed, including SA, MRSA, SE, and SIM. Of the Gram-negative bacteria detected, enteric bacteria (e.g., *Escherichia* spp.)

and several species of *Pseudomonas* were represented. In general, the veterinary clinics surveyed were largely contaminated by Gram-positive bacteria, with presumed staphylococcal contamination being the most frequent throughout the sampled sites. Notably, *S. pseudintermedius* can be problematic for both dogs and humans, possibly causing disease in both species [35]. Two of the Gram-positive rods detected, Cdiff and BAC, are spore-forming species. This is important since bacterial spores offer the species a higher degree of resistance to many abiotic factors that may be employed to control bacterial contamination. In addition, many *Bacillus* spp. are associated with soil, and since dogs are known to dig in soil quite often, veterinary patients may carry these bacteria into the clinics on their skin or feet. The other spore-forming bacteria, Cdiff, is a notable human pathogen and could pose a threat to care-giving humans in these clinics [9,10,36].

Within the clinics, several "hot spot areas" having high levels of bacterial contamination, such as HVAC return air ducts, floors, and scales, are common to veterinary patients and represent sites with which human caregivers also interact. As the results demonstrate, these areas had 50–94.7% positive swabs for multiple potential pathogenic bacteria. Of the bacteria cultured from HVAC return air ducts and from the floors, spore-forming bacteria (e.g., Cdiff and BAC) were dominant. When bacterial species that may be from soil are found on both floors and HVAC return air ducts, this suggests that levels of dust in the facilities might be high. When dust is suspended in the air, it can help transmit airborne pathogens. Airborne pathogens in human hospitals have been found to contribute to infections in both patients and their caregivers [37]. Targeted cleaning and disinfection of veterinary clinics to reduce dust may be a good strategy to reduce the potential for contamination of animals and their caregivers.

Water in the underwater treadmill tanks was contaminated by both enteric and non-specific bacteria. If the enteric bacteria observed were of fecal origin, dogs using the treadmills may be contaminated by a wide range of fecally transmitted dog pathogens [38]. One measure that can be used to reduce waterborne contamination in underwater treadmills is to use shock treatments with chlorine-, bromine-, or hydrogen peroxide-based chemical treatments. Periodic emptying of the tanks and refilling with treated water (saltwater system or low levels of bromine or chlorine) may help reduce the potential for contamination with enteric pathogens.

A recent study performed by Lord et al. found increased numbers of antimicrobial-resistant bacteria in hospitals, particularly *Staphylococcus* spp. [4]. In some cases, resistance against last-tier antimicrobial therapies (e.g., fluoroquinolones and phenicols) was observed in strains of *Staphylococcus* spp. [4,39,40]. Although methicillin-resistant *S. pseudintermedius* was not a focus of this study, it is highly probable that a horizontal exchange of resistant factors between strains of MRSA and this dog pathogen could occur [41]. Antimicrobial and multidrug-resistant pathogens are a huge public health concern to both veterinary patients and their caregivers and need to be addressed in all clinics.

This study was based on the use of viable bacterial culture techniques to monitor contamination in the veterinary clinics sampled. Many contemporary studies of the presence of bacteria (and other pathogens) in human health care facilities use some form of a molecular approach to extract DNA from samples and determine the diversity of the microorganisms present [42]. Culture techniques provide useful data with regard to the presence of viable cells on surfaces from the sampled sites. Using molecular data to describe the bacterial diversity of a site provides little or no evidence of whether the cells are viable. There is no evidence that DNA from *Staphylococcus* spp. alone causes HAIs; however, viable staphylococci could cause HAIs. Thus, the data presented here represent living contaminants present on clinical surfaces that could easily cause infections in open wounds or other sites on animal patients. Measures to address contamination in these clinics should be a priority.

Potential limiting factors related to this study fall into two areas. The first is any problems associated with the line inoculation procedure. The second is the possibility of colonial bacterial growth on the different media for species that should have been selected against, possibly confusing the identification of the species the medium is selective for. In this study, since we were only inoculating five agar-based media, we had to rotate the swab somewhere between 14% and 20% of a full rotation (see Supplementary Materials for additional details) to ensure that a fresh surface of the swab came into contact with the next agar surface being inoculated. Rotating the swabs more (or less) than that may not result in the use of a fresh swab surface to inoculate all of the media being inoculated with that swab. Another possible issue with the use of our line inoculation procedure would be the absence of colonies from a bacterial species present in very low numbers on the swab. If the numbers of this species are so low that there are not at least five cells uniformly distributed around the swab, then we may detect a species on one medium but not another in the series of media inoculated. Another concern with the use of this technique is the potential for the growth of species that may confound the identification usually made on the selective media. For example, on MSA, we know that several non-staphylococci species have been found to survive. According to the Beckton, Dickinson Co. [43] in a quality control report on their MSA medium, *Proteus mirabilis* (Gram-negative) shows "partial" growth on this medium. Another non-staphylococci species that will grow on MSA is *Bacillus subtilis*, which is tolerant of high salt concentrations. Because there are bacterial species that can grow on selective and differential media that should inhibit their growth, possible inhibition of the growth of the desired species on that medium may occur. A recent study has found that *B. subtilis* can produce a bacteriocin capable of the inhibition of *S. aureus* and some enteric bacteria [44]. If there are other such amensalistic interactions between different bacterial species on our selective and differential media, then results generated using the line inoculation procedure might miss the inhibited species. Overall, we feel that these limitations are not critical enough to change our presumptive identifications of the bacteria we identify, which should give clinic managers data to work with in their cleaning and disinfection procedures.

Areas of the veterinary clinics studied here that need to have focused cleaning and disinfection include the HVAC return air vents, scales, exercise equipment, and floors. Although ultrasound coupling gel can be obtained in sterile packets, the clinics studied use gel in reusable bottles. A previous study of human physical therapy clinic ultrasound devices found that the tips of coupling gel bottles were often contaminated with MRSA [45]. Scales are frequently used by all patients entering the clinic and increase the risk of acquiring pathogens that may result in an infection. All these factors increase the risk to veterinary patients and their human caregivers and warrant further investigation and care with disinfection.

5. Conclusions

These findings suggest that veterinary clinical environmental surfaces and water are generally contaminated by both Gram-positive and Gram-negative bacterial species. Some of the presumptive contaminating species of bacteria are known pathogens of both dogs and humans (e.g., MRSA, SA, PSA) or specifically pathogenic to humans (e.g., Cdiff). This contamination has the potential to contribute to HAIs that may occur in veterinary patients or their human caregivers. Further research is warranted to investigate the extent of bacterial contamination in veterinary clinics and any potential links to HAIs occurring in animals being treated in those clinics.

Supplementary Materials: The following supporting information can be downloaded at https://www.mdpi.com/article/10.3390/ani14131896/s1, File S1: Methods used for Presumptive Bacterial Identification Using Swabs Collected from Clinic Surfaces.

Author Contributions: Conceptualization, H.G.S. and D.L.; methodology, H.G.S.; software, D.L.; validation, N.M. and D.M.; formal analysis, H.G.S. and D.L.; investigation, H.G.S., D.L. and J.B.; resources, D.L.; data curation, H.G.S. and D.L.; writing—original draft preparation, H.G.S., D.L. and J.B.; writing—review and editing, N.M. and D.M.; visualization, H.G.S. and D.L.; supervision, H.G.S.

and D.L.; project administration, H.G.S.; funding acquisition, D.L. All authors have read and agreed to the published version of the manuscript.

Funding: This research was funded entirely by UTCs Clinical Infectious Disease Control research group, receiving no external funding.

Institutional Review Board Statement: Although this study did not involve any human or animal subjects, we were concerned that our close association with clinical environments in which animals were present in veterinary rehabilitation clinics might constitute a need to obtain approval from the University of Tennessee at Chattanooga's Institutional Animal Care and Use Committee (IACUC). We submitted a request for a review of our proposed work to UTC's IACUC on 7 February 2020. After reviewing our request, we received a letter of exemption from the IACUC on 11 February 2020, in which the committee "determined that it [this study] does not meet the threshold of research with animal subjects as defined by the United States Department of Agriculture and the Public Health Service. Therefore, your proposed activity will not require review and monitoring by the UTC IACUC".

Informed Consent Statement: Not applicable.

Data Availability Statement: We intend to make data generated in this study available via a cloud-based system provided by the University of Tennessee.

Acknowledgments: This project was funded and conducted by UTC's Clinical Infectious Disease Control research group. We would like to thank Seth LaRue for his help with estimating swab surface areas.

Conflicts of Interest: The authors declare no conflicts of interest.

References

1. Stull, J.W.; Weese, J.S. Hospital-Associated Infections in small animal practice. *Vet. Clin. N. Am. Small Anim.* **2015**, *45*, 217–233. [CrossRef] [PubMed]
2. Brigando, G.; Sutton, C.; Uebelhor, O.; Pitsoulakis, N.; Pytynia, M.; Dillon, T.; Elliott-Burke, T.; Hubert, N.; Martinez-Guryn, K.; Bolch, C.; et al. The microbiome of an outpatient rehabilitation clinic and predictors of contamination: A pilot study. *PLoS ONE* **2023**, *18*, e0281299. [CrossRef] [PubMed] [PubMed Central]
3. Kirkby, S.K.; Alvarez, L.; Foster, S.A.; Tomlinson, J.E.; Shaw, A.J.; Pozzi, A. Fundamental principles of rehabilitation and musculoskeletal tissue healing. *Vet. Surg.* **2020**, *49*, 22–32. [CrossRef] [PubMed]
4. Lord, J.; Millis, N.; Jones, R.; Johnson, B.; Kania, S.; Odoi, A. Patterns of antimicrobial, multidrug and methicillin resistance among *Staphylococcus* spp. isolated from canine specimens submitted to a diagnostic laboratory in Tennessee, USA: A descriptive study. *BMC Vet. Res.* **2022**, *18*, 91. [CrossRef] [PubMed]
5. Spratt, H., Jr.; Levine, D.; McDonald, S.; Drake, S.; Duke, K.; Kluttz, C.; Noonan, K. Survival of *Staphylococcus aureus* on therapeutic ultrasound heads. *Am. J. Infect. Control* **2019**, *47*, 1157–1159. [CrossRef] [PubMed]
6. Álvarez-Pérez, S.; Blanco, J.; Harmanus, C.; Kuijper, E.; García, M. Data from a survey of *Clostridium perfringens* and *Clostridium difficile* shedding by dogs and cats in the Madrid region (Spain), including phenotypic and genetic characteristics of recovered isolates. *Data Brief* **2017**, *14*, 88–100. [CrossRef] [PubMed] [PubMed Central]
7. Hanks, J.; Levine, D.; Bockstahler, B. Physical agent modalities in physical therapy and rehabilitation of small animals. *Vet. Clin. N. Am. Small Anim. Pract.* **2015**, *45*, 29–44. [CrossRef] [PubMed]
8. Dycus, D.L.; Levine, D.; Ratsch, B.E.; Marcellin-Little, D.J. Physical Rehabilitation for the Management of Canine Hip Dysplasia: 2021 Update. *Vet. Clin. N. Am. Small Anim. Pract.* **2022**, *52*, 719–747. [CrossRef] [PubMed]
9. Lim, S.; Knight, D.; Riley, T. *Clostridium difficile* and One Health. *Clin. Microbiol. Infect.* **2019**, *26*, 857–863. [CrossRef]
10. Alalawi, M.; Aljahdali, S.; Alharbi, B.; Fagih, L.; Fatani, R.; Aljuhani, O. *Clostridium difficile* infection in an academic medical center in Saudi Arabia: Prevalence and risk factors. *Ann. Saudi Med.* **2020**, *40*, 305–309. [CrossRef]
11. Orden, C.; Blanco, J.; Álvarez-Pérez, S.; Garcia, M.; Blanco, J.; Garcia-Sancho, M.; Rodriguez-Franco, F.; Sainz, A.; Villaescusa, A.; Harmanus, C.; et al. Isolation of *Clostridium difficile* from dogs with digestive disorders, including stable metronidazole-resistant strains. *Anaerobe* **2017**, *43*, 78–81. [CrossRef] [PubMed]
12. Rabold, D.; Espelage, W.; Sin, M.; Eckmanns, T.; Schneeberg, A.; Neubauer, H.; Mobius, N.; Hille, K.; Wieler, L.; Seyboldt, C.; et al. The zoonotic potential of *Clostridium difficile* from small companion animals and their owners. *PLoS ONE* **2018**, *13*, e0193411. [CrossRef] [PubMed]
13. Weese, J. Methicllin-Resistant *Staphylococcus aureus* in Animals. *ILAR J.* **2010**, *51*, 233–244. [CrossRef] [PubMed]
14. Morris, D.; Lautenbach, E.; Zaoutis, T.; Leckerman, K.; Edelstein, P.; Rankin, S. Potential for pet animals to harbour methicillin-resistant *Staphylococcus aureus* when residing with human MRSA patients. *Zoonoses Public Health* **2012**, *59*, 286–293. [CrossRef]
15. Worthing, K.; Brown, J.; Gerber, L.; Trott, D.; Abraham, S.; Norris, J. Methicillin-resistant staphylococci amongst veterinary personnel, personnel-owned pets, patients and the hospital environment of two small animal veterinary hospitals. *Vet. Microbiol.* **2018**, *223*, 79–85. [CrossRef]

16. Tong, S.; Davis, J.; Eichenberger, E.; Holland, T.; Fowler, V. *Staphylococcus aureus* infections: Epidemiology, pathophysiology, clinical manifestations, and management. *Clin. Microbiol. Rev.* **2015**, *28*, 603–661. [CrossRef]
17. Gómez-Sanz, E.; Torres, C.; Lozano, C.; Zarazaga, M. High diversity of *Staphylococcus aureus* and *Staphylococcus pseudintermedius* lineages and toxigenic traits in healthy pet-owning household members. Underestimating normal household contact? *Comp. Immunol. Microbiol. Infect. Dis.* **2013**, *36*, 83–94. [CrossRef] [PubMed]
18. Silva, R.; de Oliveira Júnior, C.; Blanc, D.; Pereira, S.; de Araujo, M.; Vasconcelos, A.; Lobato, F. *Clostridioides difficile* infection in dogs with chronic-recurring diarrhea responsive to dietary changes. *Anaerobe* **2018**, *51*, 50–53. [CrossRef]
19. Tomo, Y.; Sobashima, E.; Eto, H.; Yamazaki, A.; Tanegashima, K.; Edamura, K. Treatment of methicillin-resistant *Staphylococcus aureus* infection following tibial plateau leveling osteotomy in a dog. *Open Vet. J.* **2021**, *11*, 728–733. [CrossRef] [PubMed] [PubMed Central]
20. Mork, R.; Hogan, P.; Muenks, C.; Boyle, M.; Thompson, R.; Sullivan, M.; Morelli, J.; Seigel, J.; Orschein, R.; Wardenburg, J.; et al. Longitudinal, strain-specific *Staphylococcus aureus* introduction and transmission events in households of children with community-associated meticillin-resistant *S. aureus* skin and soft tissue infection: A prospective cohort study. *Lancet Infect. Dis.* **2020**, *20*, 188–198. [CrossRef]
21. Weese, J. Bacterial enteritis in dogs and cats: Diagnosis, therapy, and zoonotic potential. *Vet. Clin. N. Am. Small Anim. Pract.* **2011**, *41*, 287–309. [CrossRef] [PubMed]
22. Gingrich, E.; Kurt, T.; Hyatt, D.; Lappin, M.; Ruch-Gallie, R. Prevalence of methicillin-resistant staphylococci in northern Colorado shelter animals. *J. Vet. Diagn. Investig.* **2011**, *23*, 947–950. [CrossRef] [PubMed]
23. Nienhoff, U.; Kadlec, K.; Chaberny, I.; Verspohl, J.; Gerlach, G.-F.; Kreienbrock, L.; Schwarz, S.; Simon, D.; Nolte, I. Methicillin-resistant *Staphylococcus pseudintermedius* among dogs admitted to a small animal hospital. *Vet. Microbiol.* **2011**, *150*, 191–197. [CrossRef] [PubMed]
24. Zur, G.; Gurevich, B.; Elad, D. Prior antimicrobial use as a risk factor for resistance in selected *Staphylococcus pseudintermedius* isolates from the skin and ears of dogs. *Vet. Dermatol.* **2016**, *27*, 468-e125. [CrossRef] [PubMed]
25. Somayaji, R.; Rubin, J.; Priyantha, M.; Church, D. Exploring *Staphylococcus pseudintermedius*: An emerging zoonotic pathogen? *Future Microbiol.* **2016**, *11*, 1371–1374. [CrossRef] [PubMed]
26. Bond, R.; Loeffler, A. What's happened to *Staphylococcus intermedius*? Taxonomic revision and emergence of multi-drug resistance. *J. Small Anim. Pract.* **2012**, *53*, 147–154. [CrossRef]
27. Sasaki, T.; Kikuchi, K.; Tanaka, Y.; Takahashi, N.; Kamata, S.; Hiramatsu, K. Methicillin-resistant *Staphylococcus pseudintermedius* in a veterinary teaching hospital. *J. Clin. Microbiol.* **2007**, *45*, 1118–1125. [CrossRef]
28. Bannoehr, J.; Franco, A.; Iurescia, M.; Battisti, A.; Fitzgerald, J. Molecular diagnostic identification of *Staphylococcus pseudintermedius*. *J. Clin. Microbiol.* **2009**, *47*, 469–471. [CrossRef]
29. Bannoehr, J.; Guardabassi, L. *Staphylococcus pseudintermedius* in the dog: Taxonomy, diagnostics, ecology, epidemiology and pathogenicity. *Vet. Dermatol.* **2012**, *23*, 253-e52. [CrossRef]
30. Abouelkhair, M.; Frank, L.; Bemis, D.; Giannone, R.; Kania, S. *Staphylococcus pseudintermedius* 5'-nucleotidase suppresses canine phagocytic activity. *Vet. Microbiol.* **2020**, *246*, 108720. [CrossRef]
31. Iverson, S.; Brazil, A.; Ferguson, J.; Nelson, K.; Lautenbach, E.; Rankin, S.; Morris, D.; Davis, M. Anatomical patterns of colonization of pets with staphylococcal species in homes of people with methicillin-resistant *Staphylococcus aureus* (MRSA) skin or soft tissue infection (SSTI). *Vet. Microbiol.* **2015**, *176*, 202–208. [CrossRef] [PubMed]
32. Kmieciak, W.; Szewczyk, E. Are zoonotic Staphylococcus pseudintermedius strains a growing threat for humans? *Folia Microbiol.* **2018**, *63*, 743–747. [CrossRef] [PubMed]
33. Keilman, R.; Harding, S.; Rowin, M.; Reade, E.; Klingborg, P.; Levine, D.; Spratt, H., Jr. Investigations of Staphylococcal contamination on environmental surfaces of a neonatal intensive care unit of a children's hospital. *Am. J. Infect. Control* **2021**, *49*, 1450–1453. [CrossRef] [PubMed]
34. Flayhart, D.; Hindler, J.; Bruckner, D.; Hall, G.; Shrestha, R.; Vogel, S.; Richter, S.; Howard, W.; Walther, R.; Carroll, K. Multicenter evaluation of BBL CHROMagar MRSA medium for direct detection of methicillin-resistant *Staphylococcus aureus* from surveillance cultures of the anterior nares. *J. Clin. Microbiol.* **2005**, *43*, 5536–5540. [CrossRef] [PubMed] [PubMed Central]
35. Kelesidis, T.; Tsiodras, S. *Staphylococcus intermedius* is not only a zoonotic pathogen, but may also cause skin abscesses in humans after exposure to saliva. *Int. J. Infect. Dis.* **2010**, *14*, e838–e841. [CrossRef] [PubMed]
36. Álvarez-Pérez, S.; Blanco, J.; Harmanus, C.; Kuijper, E.; García, M. Prevalence and characteristics of Clostridium perfringens and Clostridium difficile in dogs and cats attended in diverse veterinary clinics from the Madrid region. *Anaerobe* **2017**, *48*, 47–55. [CrossRef]
37. Bonadonna, L.; Briancesco, R.; Coccia, A.; Meloni, P.; Rosa, G.; Moscato, U. Microbial Air Quality in Healthcare Facilities. *Int. J. Environ. Res. Public Health* **2021**, *18*, 6226. [CrossRef] [PubMed]
38. Murphy, C.; Reid-Smith, R.; Boerlin, P.; Weese, J.; Prescott, J.; Janecko, N.; Hassard, L.; McEwen, S. *Escherichia coli* and selected veterinary and zoonotic pathogens isolated from environmental sites in companion animal veterinary hospitals in southern Ontario. *Can. Vet. J.* **2010**, *51*, 963–972. [PubMed] [PubMed Central]
39. Mlynarczyk-Bonikowska, B.; Kowalewski, C.; Krolak-Ulinska, A.; Marusza, W. Molecular Mechanisms of Drug Resistance in *Staphylococcus aureus*. *Int. J. Mol. Sci.* **2022**, *23*, 8088. [CrossRef] [PubMed] [PubMed Central]

40. Huynh, T.Q.; Tran, V.N.; Thai, V.C.; Nguyen, H.A.; Nguyen, N.T.G.; Tran, M.K.; Nguyen, T.P.T.; Le, C.A.; Ho, L.T.N.; Surian, N.U.; et al. Genomic alterations involved in fluoroquinolone resistance development in *Staphylococcus aureus*. *PLoS ONE* **2023**, *18*, e0287973. [CrossRef]
41. Souza-Silva, T.; Rossi, C.; Andrade-Oliveira, A.; Vilar, L.; Pereira, M.; de Araujo Penna, B.; Giambiagi-deMarval, M. Interspecies transfer of plasmid-borne gentamicin resistance between *Staphylococcus* isolated from *Staphylococcus aureus*. *Infect. Genet. Evol.* **2022**, *98*, 105230. [CrossRef] [PubMed]
42. Lax, S.; Sangwan, N.; Smith, D.; Larsen, P.; Handley, K.; Richardson, M.; Guyton, K.; Krezalek, M.; Shogan, B.; Defazio, J.; et al. Bacterial colonization and succession in a newly opened hospital. *Sci. Transl. Med.* **2017**, *9*, eaah6500. [CrossRef] [PubMed]
43. Beckton, Dickinson Co. Quality Control Procedures. BBL Mannitol Salt Agar, L997389, Rev. 9 June 2017. Available online: https://static.bd.com/documents/eifu/L007389_EN.pdf (accessed on 15 June 2024).
44. Lu, Z.; Guo, W.; Liu, C. Isolation, identification and characterization of novel *Bacillus subtilis*. *J. Vet. Med. Sci.* **2018**, *80*, 427–433. [CrossRef] [PubMed]
45. Spratt, H., Jr.; Levine, D.; Tillman, L. Physical therapy clinic therapeutic ultrasound equipment as a source for bacterial contamination. *Physiother. Theory Pract.* **2014**, *30*, 507–511. [CrossRef] [PubMed]

Disclaimer/Publisher's Note: The statements, opinions and data contained in all publications are solely those of the individual author(s) and contributor(s) and not of MDPI and/or the editor(s). MDPI and/or the editor(s) disclaim responsibility for any injury to people or property resulting from any ideas, methods, instructions or products referred to in the content.

MDPI AG
Grosspeteranlage 5
4052 Basel
Switzerland
Tel.: +41 61 683 77 34

Animals Editorial Office
E-mail: animals@mdpi.com
www.mdpi.com/journal/animals

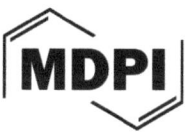

Disclaimer/Publisher's Note: The title and front matter of this reprint are at the discretion of the Guest Editors. The publisher is not responsible for their content or any associated concerns. The statements, opinions and data contained in all individual articles are solely those of the individual Editors and contributors and not of MDPI. MDPI disclaims responsibility for any injury to people or property resulting from any ideas, methods, instructions or products referred to in the content.

www.ingramcontent.com/pod-product-compliance
Lightning Source LLC
LaVergne TN
LVHW070002100526
838202LV00019B/2608